Procedures and Documentation for CT and MRI

NOTICE

Medicine is an ever-changing science. As new research and clinical experience broaden our knowledge, changes in treatment and drug therapy are required. The authors and the publisher of this work have checked with sources believed to be reliable in their efforts to provide information that is complete and generally in accord with the standards accepted at the time of publication. However, in view of the possibility of human error or changes in medical sciences, neither the authors nor the publisher nor any other party who has been involved in the preparation or publication of this work warrants that the information contained herein is in every respect accurate or complete, and they are not responsible for any errors or omissions or for the results obtained from use of such information. Readers are encouraged to confirm the information contained herein with other sources. For example and in particular, readers are advised to check the product information sheet included in the package of each drug they plan to administer to be certain that the information contained in this book is accurate and that changes have not been made in the recommended dose or in the contraindications for administration. This recommendation is of particular importance in connection with new or infrequently used drugs.

Procedures and Documentation for CT and MRI

Editor:

Roland Neseth, MS, RT, (R) (CT) (MR), RDMS
Department of Allied Health
Fort Hays State University, Hays, Kansas

Series Editor:

Erica Koch Williams, MEd, RT (R) (M) (QM)
Assistant Professor of Allied Health
Fort Hays State University, Hays, Kansas

McGraw-Hill
Medical Publishing Division

New York St. Louis San Francisco Auckland Bogotá Caracas Lisbon London Madrid Mexico City
Milan Montreal New Delhi San Juan Singapore Sydney Tokyo Toronto

12/2001

McGraw-Hill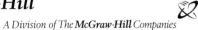

*A Division of The **McGraw·Hill** Companies*

**PROCEDURES AND DOCUMENTATION FOR
CT AND MRI**

1 2 3 4 5 6 7 8 9 0 KGP KGP 00

ISBN 0-07-135399-2

This book was set in Times Roman and Optima by V&M Graphics, Inc.
The editors were Sally Barhydt and Nicky Panton.
The production supervisor was Catherine Saggese.
Quebecor Printing/Kingsport was printer and binder.

This book is printed on acid-free paper.

Library of Congress Cataloging-in-Publication Data

Procedures and documentation for CT and MRI/editor, Roland Neseth.
    p. cm.
  ISBN 0-07-135399-2
    1. Tomography. 2. Magnetic resonance imaging. I. Neseth, Roland

  RC78.7.T6 P76 2000
  616.07′572—dc21

                                                              99-059187

Contents

Chapter 11   CT Special Procedures   **125**

Section III – Nonimaging and Quality Assurance Procedures in CT   **147**

Chapter 12   CT Experience and Patient Care   **147**

Chapter 13   **Performing Contrast Administration Procedures**   **161**

Chapter 14   **Experience Requirement for the Functions for Image Display**   **181**

Chapter 15   **Experience Requirement for Performing the Quality Assurance Procedures With the Appropriate Phantoms**   **187**

Section V – MR Imaging Procedures 221

Chapter 23 MR Imaging Procedures of the Musculosketal System **271**

Chapter 24   Advanced MR Imaging Procedures **295**

Section VI – Nonimaging and Quality Assurance Procedures in MRI **305**

Chapter 25   Intravenous Injections of Contrast Medium **305**

Preface

Written in response to the ARRT requirement for proof of clinical experience and competency prior to taking advanced imaging exams, this book addresses computed tomography (CT) and magnetic resonance imaging (MRI). Required procedures are described, and documentation pages are provided (at the back of the book). These pages can be removed from the book and sent to the ARRT when applying to take the qualifying examination.

The book continues the *Procedures and Documentation Series*, which evolved due to the current focus on competency in advanced imaging modalities. Competent CT and MRI professionals are in high demand. It is understood that keeping abreast of all protocols, equipment, and technological advances within the field is not always possible. The authors realize that institutions have specific protocol to complete certain procedures. The methods described in this text are by no means the only way to prove competency in the aforementioned fields, but instead a guide to go about documenting competency. This text should be used to supplement the clinical components of CT imaging and MRI.

A step-by-step process has been formulated for each procedure. This design should aide the professional, instructor, and student, greater ease in achieving and documenting competence in these highly technical and specialized fields.

The users are strongly encouraged to apply their knowledge and complete all requirements in order to obtain advanced qualifications in CT and MRI. While advanced qualifications do not ensure quality, they do add value to the overall knowledge of the imaging professional. Real competence can only be achieved through active participation, repetition and real interest in providing high quality care and perfecting that which one does.

Roland Neseth
Erica Koch Williams

Acknowledgments

At best, completing this book has been a challenging task that could not have been accomplished without the support of many people. I would like to thank radiographers, Daniel Hoff of St. Catherine Hospital in Garden City, Kansas, Lisa Jennison of Hays Medical Center in Hays, Kansas, and Brian Ptacek of University of Kansas Hospital in Kansas City, Kansas, for supplying the images throughout the text. My sincere gratitude goes to Mitch Weber, the Digital and Imaging Specialist at Fort Hays State University in Hays, Kansas.

Thank you to Dr. Michael Madden and Ms. Jennifer Wagner of the Department of Allied Health at Fort Hays State University. Their positive attitude and organizational skills have been a driving force for me daily. A special thanks to Ms. Erica Koch Williams who had the insight and determination to make this project a reality. I am thankful for the friendship and experiences I have shared with these people.

Thanks to my wife Cecilia, and children, Crystal and Jason, for tolerating the many frustrations and time associated with this project. Their encouragement and understanding is equally appreciated. I dedicate this book in the memory of my father, Roland Neseth. He was able to find something positive in every day, and continues to be an inspiration in my life.

In dedication to my father, Roland Neseth.

Dad, thank you for taking the time to point out the good things happening around us every day.

Roland Neseth

PART 1

CT Imaging

SECTION I

TECHNOLOGIST ASSURANCES FOR CT

CHAPTER 1

Pre-Examination Preparations

It has been said the success of the computed tomographic (CT) examination is determined before the first image ever appears on the monitor. The successful completion of the examination can be subdivided into three categories: pre-examination care, patient care, and examination imaging. The first category falls in the area of pre-examination preparation. Items in this category include a firm understanding of radiation protection, preparation of the examination room, and the selection of the proper protocol, including the selection of technical parameters.

Once the patient has arrived, the category of patient care is initiated. Patient care actually occurs before, during, and after the examination; however, in this category, the major emphasis is on the patient. The patient care category includes identification of the patient; safety screening and patient education concerning the procedure; evaluation of requisition, medical record, or both; proper documentation of patient history, including allergies; patient assessment; documentation of procedure and patient data in appropriate records. Patient care also includes the use of universal precautions, patient positioning, and discharging the patient with the appropriate instructions and precautions.

The final category of examination imaging includes image display; optimal image quality, including optimal demonstration of anatomic region; proper identification and patient data on images; image filming; and archiving; and examination completeness. It should be understood that the three categories are interdependent of one another. However, at times, each category will blend and overlap the adjacent category. Items in each category have no set order and should be considered as an overall approach to the successful completion of the

Categories of a Successful CT Imaging Procedure

Pre-examination preparation	**Examination imaging**
Radiation protection	Optimal image quality, including demonstration of anatomic region
Examination room preparation	
Selection of proper protocol, including technical parameters	Proper identification and patient data on images
	Image display, filming, and archiving
	Examination completeness
Patient care	
Identification and evaluation of the patient requisition, medical record, or both	
Documentation of patient history, including allergies	
Patient assessment	
Safety screening and patient education concerning the procedure	
Patient positioning	
Documentation of procedure and patient data into appropriate records	
Discharge the patient and inform the patient of any postprocedural instructions	
Universal precautions	

examination. The following pages will cover each category in more depth. All three categories are a critical portion of each CT imaging procedure. The technologist must be proficient in all three categories before the technologist can be recorded as competent.

A CT examination starts long before the patient arrives at the computed tomography department. This portion of the examination process deals with the pre-examination preparations necessary to ensure the efficiency of the examination.

Proper Radiation Protection

The CT technologist is responsible for the proper radiation protection for all personnel entering the CT examination room. All calibration tests and tube warm-up procedures should be performed before the patient arrives. The technologist should not leave the control room or allow anyone in the examination room during this process.

Under normal conditions, only the patient should occupy the examination room during the CT examination. There are occasions when ancillary personnel will be present during an examination. When this occurs, it is the responsibility of the technologist to provide necessary shielding equipment for all personnel present during the examination process. It should be stressed again that, under normal conditions, only the patient should be present in the examination room during radiation exposure.

Before the patient's arrival to the examination room, the technologist should prepare the room with any necessary radiation protection equipment. Because computed tomography generates images by exposing the patient to a circular pattern of radiation, it is necessary to shield the patient in all directions when applying lead shielding. Shielding the patient by placing a lead apron on top of them during scanning does very little to protect the patient when the x-ray tube is exposed from the bottom side of the gantry. Many technologists will place the first layer of shielding on the examination table and cover the shielding with a sheet or blanket before the patient arrives for the examination. After positioning the patient, the technologist will place another lead apron across the patient to provide protection from radiation exposure entering from the anterior and lateral sides of the patient. Proper shielding is an important part of the CT examination process; however, the technologist must be careful to avoid shielding the area of interest.

Preparation of Examination Room

First impressions are always important, and the preparation of the CT examination room is no different. The first thing the technologist sees in the morning is the work atmosphere. It is important to have imaging devices, quality phantoms, and the overall appearance of the work area organized for efficiency. Consistent placement of imaging items will improve the effectiveness of the technologist. First impressions are also important for the patient. The patient is often coming into an unfamiliar atmosphere when entering a computed tomography facility. For the patient, the easiest judgment comes by visually inspecting the computed tomography department. Before bringing the patient into the imaging room, it is wise for the technologist to have the room organized, including the proper imaging device such as the head holder either attached to the computed tomography unit or placed in a convenient location for the technologist when positioning the patient. Positioning sponges should be placed in an efficient yet organized location.

Selection of Proper Protocol

The proper selection of protocol is a collaborative effort between the radiologist, technologist, and manufacturer's requirements. The selection of the proper protocol is based on the idea of producing the optimal image with the least amount of radiation. The protocol will take into consideration the patient's ability to maintain the position throughout the examination, the proper gantry angulation, and acquiring the highest quality image in the least amount of time. All of the above factors should be considered on an individual basis. The manufacturer's recommendations are exactly that, "recommendations," the technologist will be responsible for determining final decisions concerned with techniques that will create the optimal image.

In addition to patient considerations, the diagnostic considerations are also a vital part in selecting the optimal imaging protocol. When selecting a protocol, it is important to place consideration to the proper technical factors that will provide optimal image quality. Technical factors such as window and level settings and reconstruction algorithms are necessary for demonstration of normal anatomy and for the visualization of pathologic conditions. The proper protocol selection will place consideration to the anatomy of interest and any anatomy or object that will generate artifacts. Artifacts from items such as dental fillings or prostheses should be imaged to reduce image artifacts as much as possible. Therefore, the proper protocol involves considerations to patients, technologists, specific anatomy, image contrast, and generation of artifacts. As with many diagnostic modalities, selection of the best protocol is a combination of balance and trade-offs between the needs of the patient, technologist, and radiologist.

Selection of Proper Imaging Parameters

Imaging parameters are often responsibilities of the manufacturer, technologist, and radiologist. There are four main factors that should be considered when determining image quality. These are signal to noise ratio, contrast to noise ratio, spatial resolution, and scan time. Often the improvement of results in one area will result in a degradation to one of the other parameters.

Signal to noise ratio (SNR) is the amount of usable signal in relationship to the amount of noise present while generating the signal. The noise of the CT system is the inherent electrical noise of the CT system components or lack of factual information. Noise is present with every examination and can vary with the area being imaged. The amount of signal can fluctuate relative to noise. Factors that increase the SNR are increasing the amount of x-ray photons detected by the image detectors, increasing pixel size, and increasing slice thickness.

Spatial resolution is the ability to distinguish two separate points of interest as two independent points of information. The points of information are displayed within the matrix of the computer monitor. The image matrix consists of picture elements or "pixels" within the field of view (FOV). The FOV is the size of the area which the pixels will be displayed. The technologist controls the size of the matrix, FOV, and therefore, the pixel size of each image. The voxel is the volume element that is the third dimension of the matrix. The slice thickness alters the voxel size. Increasing the slice thickness will increase the voxel size. Therefore, anything that affects the slice thickness, matrix size, or the number of pixels within the matrix will affect the spatial resolution of the resulting image.

The technologist should remember that the selection of slice thickness, FOV, or matrix will have a resulting effect on image quality, scan time, and quantity of examinations performed. One of the major goals of diagnostic computed tomography is to acquire a study with the highest SNR, CNR, with the highest possible spatial and contrast resolution, in the shortest amount of time. In reality, there is a constant trade-off between these parameters.

CHAPTER 2

Patient Care Preparations

This section focuses on the actual time frame when the patient is present within the imaging facility. However, patient care is a process that starts before the patient enters and continues after the patient has left the imaging facility.

Identification and Evaluation of the Patient's Requisition, Medical Record, or Both

The technologist starts the examination process before the patient physically arrives at the imaging center. Important information concerning the patient's medical needs and reason for the examination are routinely provided during the scheduling process. The technologist should ask the patient similar questions as part of the interview process to verify previous information and pertinent history. Previous diagnostic examinations should be located before the CT examination. Previous examinations are valuable for the radiologist and technologist to use as a comparative resource with current information. When there is any doubt concerning the requested examination or questions on medical history, the technologist should contact the referring physician and radiologist before examination of the patient.

Documentation of Patient History, Including Allergies

Attaining the patient history allows the technologist the opportunity to directly communicate with the patient. This process should be complete and not rushed. Many facilities use a form with questions referring to symptoms, combined with an anatomic drawing to allow the technologist and patient to mark and describe the areas of interest. Information on the history sheet should be direct and, most importantly, thorough. Questions concerning history of discomfort, previous surgeries, medications, and allergies should all be included. Patient history concerning medications and allergies is useful in the process of patient monitoring and assessment, especially when contrast medium or sedation is used for the examination. Completing the information on the questionnaire will allow the patient an opportunity to participate and allow an opportunity to increase their level of confidence in the examination process.

Patient Assessment

The technologist must reassure the patient that he or she will be monitored visually and verbally. Maintaining the patient's confidence is an important part in the successful completion of the examination process. The technologist should communicate routinely with the patient throughout the progression of the examination. With frequent communication, the technologist will notice changes in a patient's condition. Any sudden change in a patient's condition should be noted and attended to before continuing with the examination process.

Safety Screening and Patient Education Concerning the Procedure

CT uses a precise collimated beam to create images; however, this does not release the technologist from the responsibility for screening patients for potential pregnancy. During the interview process, the technologist must ascertain the patient of childbearing age is not pregnant. In the event of uncertainty, the technologist should consider the option of rescheduling the examination until proper tests are completed or confirmation of the patient's condition exists. Because of the potential risk of birth defects to the fetus, if possible, the patient should postpone the CT examination until after the first trimester. In the event that the benefits of the CT examination outweigh the risks from radiation exposure, the technologist must make a conscientious effort to properly shield the patient.

Before the CT examination, the patient should understand the reason for the examination. The patient should be informed that the examination process may include the use of oral contrast medium, which will be taken before the scan. In these cases, the patient must be informed of the importance of timing requirements and amounts of contrast medium that will be consumed. Before using intravenous contrast medium, the patient should be informed of the reason for use and precautions that accompany intravenous contrast medium. Some imaging facilities will require the patient to sign a consent form for the use of contrast agents. The technologist should understand the requirements of the imaging center.

Patient Positioning

Patient positioning is dependent on the imaging procedure, technologist, and the patient's capabilities. Manufacturers will provide guidelines for the ideal positioning for a specific examination and for their specific equipment. This information should always be considered a guideline. When the patient is unable to maintain the ideal position, the technologist has the option to alter the position or not complete the examination. Rarely is the latter the only option. Normal imaging of the head, neck, cervical spine, thoracic spine, or a combination of the whole spine, shoulders, chest, and abdomen is completed with the patient placed head first in the CT scanner. Imaging of the lower extremities and lumbar spine is completed with the patient entering the CT scanner feet first. The chapter containing the imaging procedures is based on a blend of technologist's preference, radiologist's preference, and manufacturer's recommendations. Procedures will frequently be adjusted to serve the patient as well as the technologist's and radiologist's needs. The procedures in the following chapters are to be used strictly as guidelines.

In addition, to physically position the patient according to the examination protocol, it is wise to make sure the patient is comfortable before acquiring images. This is done by using any combination of positioning sponges, blankets, and restraining devices. The time spent making the patient comfortable will be returned through patient cooperation and reduction of patient motion.

Documentation of Procedure and Patient Data in Appropriate Records

During the actual examination, it is important to complete the proper documentation of the examination process. Many CT imaging facilities keep a log book for storing the statistical information of the specific examination. Information should include patient, contrast, and scan information. Any negative reaction that occurred during the examination should be noted in the log book.

Discharge the Patient and Inform the Patient of Any Postprocedural Instructions

After the successful completion of the CT examination, removal of all positioning sponges and restraining devices is necessary. The patient should be allowed a moment to reorient to the setting before leaving the examination table. The technologist should inform the patient on the approximate time regarding the results of the examination and any possible side effects from oral or intravenous contrast medium.

Universal Precautions

Universal precautions are always important when working with patients. These precautions are designed to protect health care workers from bloodborne pathogens. It is common practice to use universal precautions consistently for every patient the technologist is in contact. There should be a standard use of gloves when in contact with blood, bodily fluids, or nonintact skin. The use of gowns and protective eyewear may be necessary to complete a procedure that may involve blood or bodily fluids. Gowns should be removed after saturation or completion of examination. Needles should be properly disposed of upon completion of use. After completion of the examination, the technologist should properly wash his or her hands. Each imaging facility should have a complete list of universal precautions to use as a reference. The technologist should understand and be able to perform universal precautions before performing examinations on patients.

CHAPTER 3

Examination Imaging Category

Image quality must be evaluated daily; this evaluation is done with the help of CT quality phantoms. The quality tests should be completed consistently as part of the morning routine for the technologist. Results of the quality test should be stored for the required time and act as a reference to subtle changes within image quality. In addition to routine quality testing, the technologist should visually inspect the quality of each image produced during the CT examination.

Optimal Image Quality, Including Demonstration of Anatomic Region

The quality of the examination is dependent on the diagnostic value of the images created. The optimal study will contain a combination of the best possible signal to noise ratio (SNR), contrast to noise ratio (CNR), and spatial resolution which are completed in a reasonable amount of time. The resulting image should display the appropriate anatomy with the proper image weighting applied. The technologist should be aware that the idealistic belief of attaining the optimal level of each parameter is not possible. Therefore, the technologist must determine which areas need to be optimal and the levels of acceptability. Normally, the quality of the image will supersede the importance of speed. The quality of an image should be reproducible and consistent through a variety of examinations and patients.

Proper Identification and Patient Data on Images

Each image should have the proper patient identification present. The information must be correct and current for the patient. Proper use of patient and facility data should be consistent on each sheet of images. Additional patient data and scan information are displayed according to radiologist's preference and standards associated with the imaging center. Some imaging centers routinely place an abbreviated version of patient history and scan data on each image.

Image Display, Filming, and Archiving

The optimal study will include the appropriate imaging planes and technical parameters preferred by the imaging center. This means each image will display the appropriate field of view, proper slice thicknesses, images will be free of motion, and have the proper annotation on each film. Upon completion of the examination, the technologist should record the images to the preferred filming format. This includes the scan information menu and images in the preferred sequence. The technologist should inspect the processed films for appropriate quality. After the successful filming of the study, the technologist should save the examination information on the proper data storage system. The data are to be stored for the length of time required by the imaging facility.

Examination Completeness

Upon the successful completion of the examination process and after the dismissal of the patient, the technologist should prepare the CT imaging room for the next examination. The examination room should have the bedding replaced, positioning sponges and anatomic holders stored in the proper location, and any contrast or injection materials should be removed and disposed of in the proper location. The past films, current films, and current patient history are collected and ready for the radiologist to view the study. The technologist is now ready to prepare the examination room for the next patient.

CT IMAGING PROCEDURES

CHAPTER 4

CT Imaging Procedures of the Head

The protocol marked with an asterisk must be completed on a patient, not a simulation.

	Mandatory	Elective
Head		
Routine brain*	10*	
Temporal bones	5	
Pituitary		3
Orbit	5	
Sinuses	5	
Maxillofacial	5	
Temporomandibular joint		3
Cerebral angiography		3

CT EXAMINATION OF THE BRAIN

Mandatory minimum required is 10. This protocol must be completed on a patient and not a simulation.

Common Indications

- Trauma
- Evaluation of tumors and vascular lesions
- Disruption of the blood-brain barrier
- Congenital concerns
- Inflammatory disease

Imaging Considerations

CT imaging of the brain optimally is completed with and without intravenous contrast enhancement. The noncontrast study of the brain is completed before the intravenous injection of contrast medium. Contrast injections are sometimes contraindicated for physiologic reasons such as cerebral trauma and aneurysms. The technologist should be aware of all contraindications for the use of contrast medium before the examination of every patient. The type of contrast and dosage to be used is determined by the facility requirements and manufacturer's recommendations.

Upon completion of the noncontrast examination, the technologist should change the image annotation to demonstrate the injection of contrast medium. When using intravenous contrast medium for imaging of the brain, the technologist should inject the total amount of contrast medium before resuming scanning. The same patient position and both ranges of slices are similar for the second procedure.

When imaging, the technologist should match the appropriate field of view (FOV) with the patient. The decision to use conventional or spiral scanning is determined by the imaging facility and with consideration to the patient's ability to remain motionless during the examination. An accurate explanation of the examination process and consideration of patient comfort will reduce voluntary motion during the imaging process.

Patient Preparations

The patient is placed supine and head first on the examination table. The head is hyperextended and placed in the head holder. The head is positioned with the midsagittal plane of the patient parallel with the longitudinal positioning light. The interpupillary line is parallel with the horizontal positioning lights. The technologist should use positioning pads and restraining straps as needed. The patient's arms should be placed across the abdomen or at the sides of the patient. To minimize motion artifacts, the use of restraining straps across the patient's forehead, chin, or both, should be considered. Foam padding placed under the patient's knees can relieve pressure on the lower back and add to the patient's comfort, which reduces the likelihood of patient motion. Thorough but simple instructions involving the imaging procedure will also reduce patient motion. Proper placement of radiation shielding is also an essential part of every CT examination.

Imaging Protocols

The first image produced is the lateral head. From the scout image, the technologist normally selects two imaging ranges. The first range is from the base of the skull through the petrous pyramids. The second range of slices will be from the end of the first range and

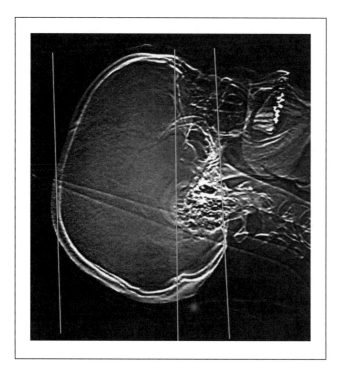

FIGURE 4-1

Lateral view of head with two axial ranges.

extending to the superior aspect of the brain tissue. The slice thickness in the first range is normally thinner in comparison to the second range, to accommodate for artifacts created by the petrous pyramids. Angulation of axial slices is often determined by radiologist preference. Certain facilities require the axial slices to be angled parallel with the orbitomeatal line, whereas other facilities prefer an angulation of 15° superior to the orbitomeatal lines. One of the benefits of angulation is to reduce the radiation dose to the patient's eyes and improve visualization of the posterior fossa (Fig. 4-1).

CT EXAMINATION OF THE TEMPORAL BONES

Mandatory minimum required is 5.

Common Indications

- Evaluation of ossicle and structures along the medial wall of the ear
- Detection of lesions in the supratentorial or infratentorial location
- Cholesteatoma of the middle ear
- Aids in the planning of neurosurgery

Imaging Considerations

Temporal bones are normally scanned in both axial and coronal planes. Axial scanning is similar to brain scanning. The FOV for axial and coronal images should display both temporal bones simultaneously. Slices within the range are normally thin to improve image quality and compensate for differing densities within the temporal bones. The range of axial images should be generated from the inferior aspect of the skull through the petrous pyramids. The coronal images should be perpendicular to the axial images. When scanning in the coronal plane, the scan FOV should include both temporal bones. After the examination, the bones may be demonstrated individually in their own FOV. The choice of conventional scanning or spiral scanning is determined by the imaging facility. An accurate explanation of the examination process, including the different patient positions, will improve patient comfort and will reduce voluntary motion during the imaging process. Contrast medium should be used per facility standards.

Patient Preparations

AXIAL IMAGES OF THE TEMPORAL BONES

The patient is placed supine and head first on the examination table. The head is hyperextended and placed in the head holder. The head is positioned with the midsagittal plane of the patient parallel with the longitudinal positioning light. The interpupillary line is parallel with the horizontal positioning lights. The technologist should use positioning pads and restraining straps as needed. The patient's arms should be placed across the abdomen or at the sides of the patient. To minimize motion artifacts, the use of restraining straps across the patient's forehead, chin, or both, should be considered. Foam padding placed under the patient's knees can relieve pressure on the lower back and add to the patient's comfort, which reduces the likelihood of patient motion. Thorough but simple instructions involving the imaging procedure will also reduce patient motion. Proper placement of radiation shielding is also an essential part of every CT examination.

Imaging Protocols

AXIAL IMAGES OF THE TEMPORAL BONES

The first image produced is of the lateral head. From the scout image, the technologist normally selects two imaging ranges. The scan range is from the base of the skull through the petrous pyramids. Thin slices are usually selected to accommodate for artifacts created by the petrous pyramids. Angulation of axial slices is often determined by

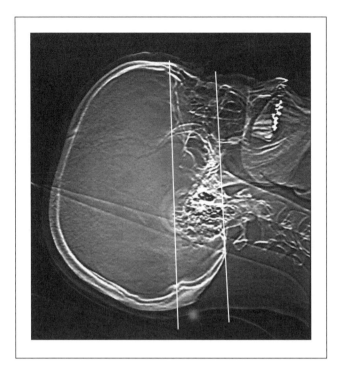

FIGURE 4-2

Lateral view of the temporal bones with axial slices from the base of the skull through the petrous pyramids.

radiologist preference. Certain facilities require the axial slices to be angled parallel with the orbitomeatal line, whereas other facilities prefer an angulation of 15° superior to the orbitomeatal lines. One of the benefits of angulation is the reduction of radiation dose to the patient's eyes (Fig. 4-2).

Patient Preparations

CORONAL IMAGES OF THE TEMPORAL BONES

The patient is placed prone and head first on the examination table. The head is hyperextended and placed in the head holder. Position the patient's head with the midsagittal plane of the patient parallel with the longitudinal positioning light. The interpupillary line should be parallel with the horizontal positioning light. The technologist should use positioning pads and restraining straps as needed. The patient's arms should be placed along the sides or underneath the patient. To minimize motion artifacts, the use of restraining straps across the posterior portion of the neck or skull should be considered. Foam padding placed under the anterior surface of the patient's lower legs can relieve pressure on the lower legs and add to the patient's comfort, which reduces the likelihood of patient motion.

If the patient is unable to hyperextend the neck while in the prone position, the technologist may consider a supine approach in patient positioning. When positioning the patient for a supine approach, the technologist should elevate the patient's lower back and buttock

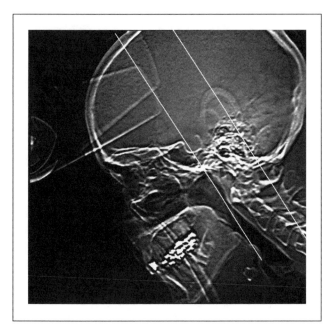

FIGURE 4-3

Demonstration of the coronal scan range extending from the point 2 cm anterior to the external auditory meatus to 1 cm posterior to the external auditory meatus.

region with appropriate padding. The technologist should adjust the head support to accommodate the supine position. Thorough but simple instructions involving the imaging procedure will also reduce patient motion. Proper placement of radiation shielding is also an essential part of every CT examination.

Imaging Protocols

CORONAL IMAGES OF THE TEMPORAL BONES

The first image produced is the lateral head. From the scout image, the technologist normally selects the imaging range. The range is from the point approximately 2 cm anterior to the external auditory meatus to point 1 cm posterior to the external auditory meatus. The coronal images should be perpendicular to the axial slices. To compensate for the angulation, the CT gantry may need to be tilted to the appropriate angle. The slice thickness is thin to accommodate for artifacts created by the petrous pyramids as well as improvement of spatial resolution and reduction of volume imaging (Fig. 4-3).

CT EXAMINATION OF THE PITUITARY

Elective minimum required is 3.

Common Indications

- Evaluation of pituitary and parasellar masses

Imaging Considerations

Pituitary scans are normally completed with contrast enhancement. The pituitary study typically requires both axial and coronal imaging. The FOV for axial and coronal images should display the lateral borders of the skull simultaneously. The slices within the scan range of both coronal and axial images are normally thin to improve image quality and compensate for differing densities within the temporal bones. The range of axial images should be generated from the roof of the sphenoid sinus through the dorsum sella. The coronal images should be perpendicular to the axial images. When scanning in the coronal plane, the scan FOV should include both temporal bones. The range of coronal slices should extend from the anterior clinoid through the dorsum sella.

Contrast medium is routinely used to enhance pituitary and parasellar masses. Contrast medium should be used according to radiologist and facility standards. The decision to use conventional scanning or spiral scanning is determined by the imaging facility and with consideration to the patient's ability to remain motionless during the examination. An accurate explanation of the examination process and consideration of patient comfort will reduce voluntary motion during the imaging process. The technologist should remember that the proper placement of radiation shielding is also an essential part of every CT examination.

Patient Preparations

AXIAL IMAGES OF THE PITUITARY

The patient is placed supine and head first on the examination table. The head is hyperextended and placed in the head holder. The patient's head is positioned with the midsagittal plane parallel with the longitudinal positioning light. The interpupillary line is parallel with the horizontal positioning lights. The technologist should use positioning pads and restraining straps as needed. The patient's arms should be placed across the abdomen or along the sides. To reduce motion artifacts, the use of restraining straps across the patient's forehead, chin, or both, should be considered. Foam padding placed under the patient's knees can relieve pressure on the lower back and add to the patient's comfort, which reduces the likelihood of patient motion. Thorough but simple instructions involving the imaging procedure will also reduce patient motion. The technologist should remember that the proper placement of radiation shielding is also an essential part of every CT examination.

Imaging Protocols

AXIAL IMAGES OF THE PITUITARY

The first image produced is the lateral head. From the scout image, the technologist normally selects the imaging range. The range is from the roof of the sphenoid sinus to the dorsum sella. Thin slices are usually selected to accommodate for artifacts created by the petrous pyramids and improve spatial resolution. Angulation of axial slices is often determined by radiologist preference. Certain facilities require the axial slices to be angled parallel with the orbitomeatal line, whereas other facilities prefer an angulation of 15° superior to the orbitomeatal lines. One of the benefits of angulation is the reduction in radiation dose to the patient's eyes (Fig. 4-4).

Patient Preparations

CORONAL IMAGES OF THE PITUITARY

The patient is placed prone and head first on the examination table. The head is hyperextended and placed in the head holder. The patient's head is positioned with the midsagittal plane parallel with the longitudinal positioning light. The interpupillary line is parallel with the horizontal positioning lights. The technologist should use positioning pads and restraining straps as needed. The patient's arms should be placed along the sides. To reduce motion artifacts, the use of restraining straps across the posterior portion of the neck or

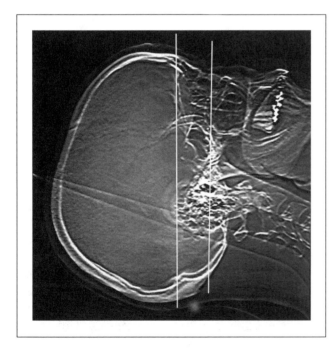

FIGURE 4-4

Lateral view of the pituitary with angled slices from the roof of the sphenoid sinus to the dorsum sella.

skull should be considered. Foam padding placed under the anterior surface of the patient's lower legs can relieve pressure on the lower legs and add to the patient's comfort.

If the patient is unable to hyperextend the neck while in the prone position, the technologist may consider a supine approach in patient positioning. When positioning the patient for a supine approach, the technologist should elevate the patient's lower back and buttock region with appropriate padding. The technologist should adjust the head support to accommodate the supine position. Thorough but simple instructions involving the imaging procedure will also reduce patient motion. The technologist should remember that the proper placement of radiation shielding is also an essential part of every CT examination

Imaging Protocols

CORONAL IMAGES OF THE PITUITARY

The first image produced is the lateral head. From the scout image, the technologist normally selects the coronal imaging range. The range is from the anterior clinoid through the dorsum sella. The coronal images should be perpendicular to the axial slices. To compensate for the angulation, the CT gantry may need to be tilted to the appropriate angle. The slice thickness is thin to improve spatial resolution and reduce volume averaging (Fig. 4-5).

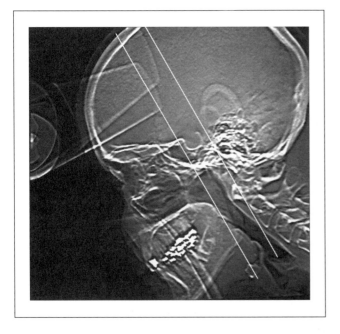

FIGURE 4-5

Lateral view of the pituitary with coronal range extending from the anterior clinoid through the dorsum sella.

CT EXAMINATION OF THE ORBIT

Mandatory minimum required is 5.

Common Indications

- Evaluation of orbital rectus muscles
- Evaluation of optic nerve

Imaging Considerations

Imaging of the orbits is completed with both axial and coronal images. For axial images, the FOV should display both lateral borders of the skull, with the anterior border extending from the globe through the dorsum sella posteriorly. The slices within the scan range of both coronal and axial images are normally thin to improve image quality. The range of axial images should be generated from the superior border of the maxillary sinus through the superior orbital rim.

The coronal images should be perpendicular to the axial images. When scanning in the coronal plane, the scan FOV should include both orbits simultaneously. The range of coronal slices should extend from the anterior border of the globe through the sphenoid sinus. Contrast medium is often used when neoplasm or vascular abnormalities are suspected. Contrast medium should be used according to facility standards. The decision to use conventional scanning or spiral scanning is determined by the imaging facility and with consideration to the patient's ability to remain motionless during the examination. Before the examination, an accurate explanation of the examination process, including the different patient positions, will improve patient comfort and will reduce voluntary motion during the imaging process.

Patient Preparations

Axial Images of the Orbits

The patient is placed supine and head first on the examination table. The head is hyperextended and placed in the head holder. The head is positioned with the midsagittal plane parallel with the longitudinal positioning light. The interpupillary line is parallel with the horizontal positioning lights. The technologist should use positioning pads and restraining straps as needed. The patient's arms should be placed across the abdomen or along the sides. To minimize motion artifacts, the use of restraining straps across the patient's forehead, chin, or both, should be considered. Foam padding placed under the patient's knees can relieve pressure on the lower back and add to the patient's comfort. Thorough but simple instructions involving the imaging procedure will also reduce patient motion. Another method to reduce motion artifacts generated by the rectus muscles is to instruct the patient to focus the eyes upward such as at a point on the top of the gantry. The technologist should remember that the proper placement of radiation shielding is also an essential part of every CT examination.

Imaging Protocols

AXIAL IMAGES OF THE ORBITS

The first image produced is the lateral head. From the scout image, the technologist normally selects the imaging range. The range is from the superior border of the maxillary sinus through the superior orbital rim. Thin slices are usually selected to accommodate for artifacts created by the petrous pyramids and improve spatial resolution. The FOV should be large enough to accommodate the lateral borders of both orbits. Angulation of axial slices is often determined by radiologist preference. For specific imaging of the optic canal, the technologist should adjust the angulation of the axial slices to a parallel line extending from the infraorbital border to the anterior clinoid. This ranges of slices should extend through the superior orbital rim (Figs. 4-6 and 4-7).

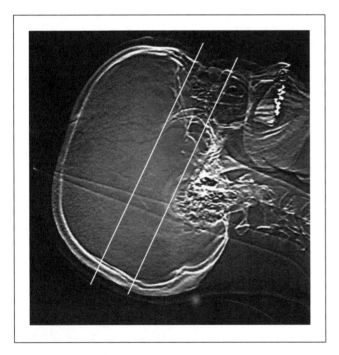

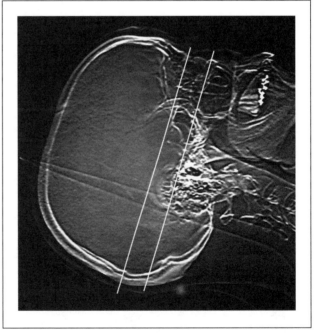

FIGURE 4-6

Lateral view of the orbits with axial slices from the superior border of the maxillary sinus through the superior orbital rim.

FIGURE 4-7

Lateral view of the orbits with axial slices from a line extending from the infraorbital border to the anterior clinoid.

Patient Preparations

CORONAL IMAGES OF THE ORBITS

The patient is placed prone and head first on the examination table. The head is hyperextended and placed in the head holder. The head is positioned with the midsagittal plane parallel with the longitudinal positioning light. The interpupillary line is parallel with the horizontal positioning lights. The technologist should use positioning pads and restraining straps as needed. The patient's arms should be placed along the sides of the patient. To minimize motion artifacts, the use of restraining straps across the posterior portion of the neck or skull should be considered. Foam padding placed under the anterior surface of the patient's lower legs can relieve pressure on the lower legs and add to the patient's comfort.

If the patient is unable to hyperextend the neck while in the prone position, the technologist may consider a supine approach in patient positioning. When positioning the patient for a supine approach, the technologist should elevate the patient's lower back and buttock region with appropriate padding. The technologist should adjust the head support to accommodate the supine position. Thorough but simple instructions involving the imaging procedure will also reduce patient motion. Proper placement of radiation shielding is also an essential part of every CT examination.

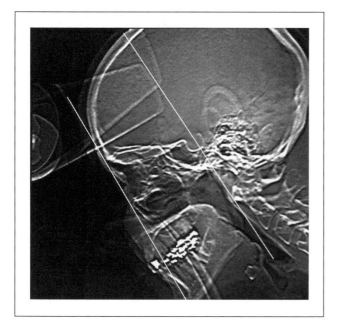

FIGURE 4-8

Lateral view of the orbit with coronal scan range extending from the sphenoid sinus to the anterior globe.

Imaging Protocols

CORONAL IMAGES OF THE ORBITS

The first image produced is the lateral head. From the scout image, the technologist normally selects the coronal imaging range. The range is from the sphenoid sinus to the anterior border of the globe. The images should be perpendicular to the axial slices. To compensate for the angulation, the CT gantry may need to be tilted to the appropriate angle. The slice thickness is thin to improve spatial resolution and reduce volume averaging. The FOV should be large enough to accommodate the lateral borders of both orbits (Fig. 4-8).

CT EXAMINATION OF THE PARANASAL SINUSES

Mandatory minimum required is 5.

Common Indications

- Evaluation of neoplasms and vascular abnormalities
- Sinusitis
- Demonstration of traumatic or pathologic bone destruction

Imaging Considerations

Imaging of the paranasal sinuses is best demonstrated with coronal images; however, axial images are also included in the typical CT examination of the sinuses. For coronal images, the FOV should display both lateral borders of the skull, as well as the superior border of the frontal bone and inferior border of the hard palate. The slices within the scan range of both coronal and axial images are normally thin to improve spatial resolution. The axial images should be perpendicular to the coronal images. The FOV for axial and coronal images should be large enough to accommodate the lateral borders of the temporal bones. Contrast medium can be used in cases of suspected neoplasm and vascular abnormalities. However, contrast medium is normally not used when evaluating the patient for sinusitis. Contrast medium should be used according to the facility standards. An accurate explanation of the examination process, including the different patient positions, will improve patient comfort and will reduce voluntary motion during the imaging process. The decision to use conventional scanning or spiral scanning is determined by the imaging facility and with consideration to the patient's ability to remain motionless during the examination.

Patient Preparations

AXIAL IMAGES OF THE PARANASAL SINUSES

The patient is placed supine and head first on the examination table. The head is hyperextended and placed in the head holder. The head is positioned with the midsagittal plane parallel with the longitudinal positioning lights. The interpupillary line is parallel with the horizontal positioning lights. The technologist should use positioning pads and restraining straps as needed. The patient's arms should be placed across the abdomen or along the sides. To minimize motion artifacts, the use of restraining straps across the patient's forehead, chin, or both, should be considered. Foam padding placed under the patient's knees can relieve pressure on the lower back and add to the patient's comfort, which reduces the likelihood of patient motion. Thorough but simple instructions involving the imaging procedure will also reduce patient motion. The technologist should remember that the proper placement of radiation shielding is also an essential part of every CT examination.

Imaging Protocols

AXIAL IMAGES OF THE PARANASAL SINUSES

The first image produced is of the lateral head. From the scout image, the technologist normally selects the imaging range. The range is from the inferior border of the hard palate through the superior border of the frontal sinuses. Thin slices are usually selected to accommodate for artifacts created by the petrous pyramids and improve spatial resolution. The FOV should be large enough to accommodate the lateral borders of the skull. Angulation of axial slices is often determined by the radiologist's preference. Certain facilities require the axial slices to be angled parallel with the orbitomeatal line, whereas other facilities prefer an angulation of 15° superior to the orbitomeatal lines (Fig. 4-9).

Patient Preparations

CORONAL IMAGES OF THE PARANASAL SINUSES

The patient is placed prone and head first on the examination table. The head is hyperextended and placed in the head holder. The patient's head is positioned with the midsagittal plane parallel with the longitudinal positioning lights. The interpupillary line is parallel with the horizontal positioning lights. The technologist should use positioning pads and restraining straps as needed. The patient's arms should be placed along the sides of the patient. To minimize motion artifacts, the use of restraining straps across the posterior portion of the neck or skull should be considered.

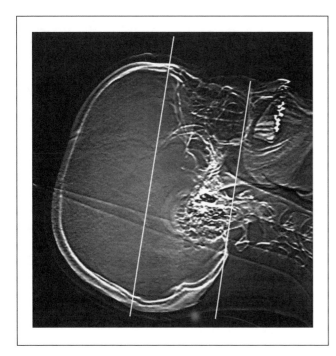

FIGURE 4-9

Lateral view of sinuses with axial slices from the inferior border of the hard palate through the superior border of the frontal sinus.

Foam padding placed under the anterior surface of the patient's lower legs can relieve pressure on the lower legs and add to the patient's comfort.

If the patient is unable to hyperextend the neck while in the prone position, the technologist may consider a supine approach in patient positioning. When positioning the patient for a supine approach, the technologist should elevate the patient's lower back and buttock region with appropriate padding. The technologist should adjust the head support to accommodate the supine position. Thorough but simple instructions involving the imaging procedure will also reduce patient motion. The technologist should remember that the proper placement of radiation shielding is also an essential part of every CT examination.

Imaging Protocols

CORONAL IMAGES OF THE PARANASAL SINUSES

The first image produced is of the lateral head. From the scout image, the technologist normally selects the coronal imaging range. The range is from the anterior border of the frontal sinus through the dorsum sella. The coronal images should be perpendicular to the axial slices. To compensate for the angulation, the CT gantry may need to be tilted to the appropriate angle. The slice thickness is thin to improve spatial resolution and reduce volume averaging. The FOV should be large enough to accommodate the lateral borders of the skull (Fig. 4-10).

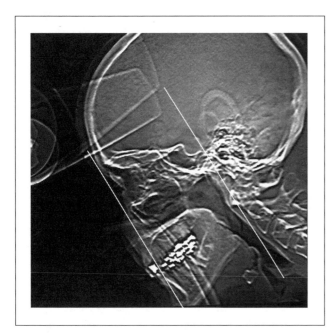

FIGURE 4-10

Lateral view of the sinus with coronal range extending from the anterior border of the frontal bone through the dorsum sella.

CT EXAMINATION OF THE MAXILLOFACIAL BONES

Mandatory minimum required is 5.

Common Indications

- Demonstration of facial bones
- Head trauma
- Demonstration of pathologic bone destruction

Imaging Considerations

Imaging of the maxillofacial bones is typically demonstrated in both coronal and axial images. For coronal images, the FOV should display both lateral borders of the skull, as well as the superior border of the frontal bone and inferior border of the hard palate. The axial images should be perpendicular to the coronal images. The FOV for axial and coronal images should be large enough to accommodate the lateral borders of the temporal bones. The slices within the scan range of both coronal and axial images are normally thin to improve spatial resolution. Contrast medium can be used in cases of suspected neoplasm and vascular abnormalities. However, contrast medium is normally not used when evaluating the patient after trauma to the facial bones. Contrast medium should be used according to facility standards. An accurate explanation of the examination process, including the different patient positions, will improve patient comfort and will reduce voluntary motion during the imaging process. The decision to use conventional scanning or spiral scanning is determined by the imaging facility and with consideration to the patient's ability to remain motionless during the examination. In cases of trauma to the maxillofacial bones, the technologist may consider 3D reconstructions to assist for surgical evaluation.

Patient Preparations

AXIAL IMAGES OF THE MAXILLOFACIAL BONES

The patient is placed supine and head first on the examination table. The head is hyperextended and placed in the head holder. Position the patient's head with the midsagittal plane parallel with the longitudinal positioning lights. The interpupillary line is parallel with the horizontal positioning light. The technologist should use positioning pads and restraining straps as needed. The patient's arms should be placed across the abdomen or along the sides. To minimize motion artifacts, the use of restraining straps across the patient's forehead, chin, or both, should be considered. Foam padding placed under the patient's knees can relieve pressure on the lower back and add to the patient's comfort, which reduces the likelihood of patient motion. Thorough but simple instructions involving the imaging procedure will also reduce patient motion. Proper placement of radiation shielding is also an essential part of every CT examination.

Imaging Protocols

AXIAL IMAGES OF THE MAXILLOFACIAL BONES

The first image produced is the lateral head. From the scout image, the technologist normally selects the axial imaging range. The range is from the inferior border of the hard palate through the superior border of the cranium. Thin slices are usually selected to accommodate for artifacts created by the petrous pyramids and improve spatial resolution. For axial images, the FOV should be large enough to accommodate the lateral borders of the temporal bones and the anterior border of the nose. Angulation of axial slices is often determined by the radiologist's preference. Certain facilities require the axial slices to be angled parallel with the orbitomeatal line, whereas other facilities prefer an angulation of 15° superior to the orbitomeatal lines (Fig. 4-11).

Patient Preparations

CORONAL IMAGES OF THE MAXILLOFACIAL BONES

The patient is placed prone and head first on the examination table. The head is hyperextended and placed in the head holder. Position the patient's head with the midsagittal plane parallel with the longitudinal positioning light. The interpupillary line is parallel

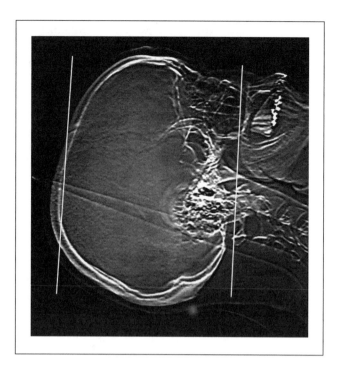

FIGURE 4-11

Lateral view of the maxillofacial bones with axial slices from the inferior border of the hard palate through the superior border of the cranium.

with the horizontal positioning lights. The technologist should use positioning pads and restraining straps as needed. The patient's arms should be placed along the sides of the patient. To minimize motion artifacts, the use of restraining straps across the posterior portion of the neck or skull should be considered. Foam padding placed under the anterior surface of the patient's lower legs can relieve pressure on the lower legs and add to the patient's comfort, which reduces the likelihood of patient motion.

If the patient is unable to hyperextend the neck while in the prone position, the technologist may consider a supine approach in patient positioning. When positioning the patient for a supine approach, the technologist should elevate the patient's lower back and buttock region with appropriate padding. The technologist should adjust the head support to accommodate the supine position. Thorough but simple instructions involving the imaging procedure will also reduce patient motion. The technologist should remember that the proper placement of radiation shielding is also an essential part of every CT examination.

Imaging Protocols

CORONAL IMAGES OF THE MAXILLOFACIAL BONES

The first image produced is of the lateral head. From the scout image, the technologist normally selects the coronal imaging range. The FOV should include the superior border of the frontal bone and the inferior border of the hard palate. The range is from the anterior border of the orbits through the dorsum sella. The coronal images

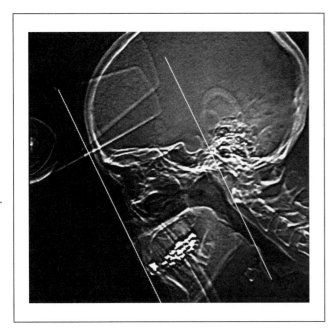

FIGURE 4-12

Lateral view of the maxillofacial bones with coronal range extending from the anterior border of the orbits through the dorsum sella.

should be perpendicular to the axial slices. To compensate for the angulation, the CT gantry may need to be tilted to the appropriate angle. The slice thickness is thin to improve spatial resolution and reduce volume averaging (Fig. 4-12).

CT EXAMINATION OF THE TEMPOROMANDIBULAR JOINT

Elective minimum required is 3.

Common Indications

- Evaluation of the relationship between the mandibular condyle and temporal bone

Imaging Considerations

Imaging of the temporomandibular joint (TMJ) is typically demonstrated in both coronal and axial images. For coronal images, the FOV should display both lateral borders of the skull, as well as the superior border of the frontal bone and inferior border of the hard palate. The slices within the scan range of both coronal and axial images are normally thin to improve spatial resolution. The axial images should be perpendicular to the coronal images. The FOV for axial and coronal images should be large enough to include both lateral borders of the temporal bones. Contrast medium is typically not used for the examination of the TMJs. Before the examination, an accurate explanation of the examination process, including the different patient positions, will improve patient comfort and will reduce voluntary motion during the imaging process. The decision to use conventional scanning or spiral scanning is determined by the imaging facility and with consideration to the patient's ability to remain motionless during the examination.

Patient Preparations

AXIAL IMAGES OF THE TEMPOROMANDIBULAR JOINT

The patient is placed supine and head first on the examination table. The head is hyperextended and placed in the head holder. The patient's head is positioned with the midsagittal plane parallel with the longitudinal positioning light. The interpupillary line is parallel with the horizontal positioning lights. The technologist should use positioning pads and restraining straps as needed. The patient's arms should be placed across the abdomen or along the sides. To minimize motion artifacts, the use of restraining straps across the patient's forehead, chin, or both, should be considered. Foam padding placed under the patient's knees can relieve pressure on the lower back and add to the patient's comfort, which reduces the likelihood of patient motion. Thorough but simple instructions involving the imaging procedure will also reduce patient motion.

Imaging Protocols

AXIAL IMAGES OF THE TEMPOROMANDIBULAR JOINT

The first image produced is the lateral head. From the scout image, the technologist normally selects the axial imaging range. The range is from the inferior border of the mandibular condyle through the mandibular fossa. Thin slices are usually selected to improve spatial resolution. The FOV should be large enough to accommodate the lateral borders of the skull. Angulation of axial slices is often determined by the radiologist's preference. Axial slices are typically angled parallel with the orbitomeatal line (Fig. 4-13).

Patient Preparations

CORONAL IMAGES OF THE TEMPOROMANDIBULAR JOINT

The patient is placed prone and head first on the examination table. The head is hyperextended and placed in the head holder. The patient's head is positioned with the midsagittal plane parallel with the longitudinal positioning light. The interpupillary line is parallel with the horizontal positioning lights. The technologist should use positioning pads and restraining straps as needed. The

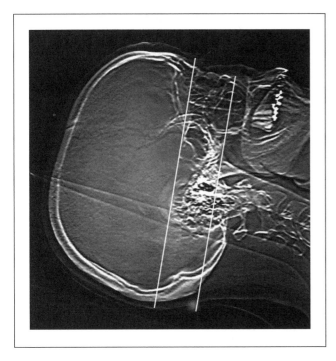

FIGURE 4-13

Lateral view of the temporomandibular joints with axial slices from the inferior border of the mandibular condyle through the mandibular fossa.

patient's arms should be placed along the sides. To minimize motion artifacts, the use of restraining straps across the posterior portion of the neck or skull should be considered. Foam padding placed under the anterior surface of the patient's lower legs can relieve pressure on the lower legs and add to the patient's comfort, which reduces the likelihood of patient motion.

If the patient is unable to hyperextend the neck while in the prone position, the technologist may consider a supine approach in patient positioning. When positioning the patient for a supine approach, the technologist should elevate the patient's lower back and buttock region with appropriate padding. The technologist should adjust the head support to accommodate the supine position. Thorough but simple instructions involving the imaging procedure will also reduce patient motion. The technologist should remember that the proper placement of radiation shielding is also an essential part of every CT examination.

Imaging Protocols

Coronal Images of the Temporomandibular Joint

The first image produced is of the lateral head. From the scout image, the technologist normally selects the coronal imaging range. The range is from slightly anterior to the mandibular condyle extending through the posterior border of the mandibular condyle. The images should be perpendicular to the axial slices. To compensate for

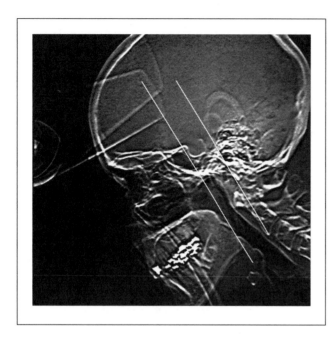

FIGURE 4-14

Lateral view of the temporomandibular joint with coronal range extending from slightly anterior to the mandibular condyle through the posterior border of the mandibular condyle.

the angulation, the CT gantry may need to be tilted to the appropriate angle. The slice thickness is thin to improve spatial resolution and reduce volume averaging (Fig. 4-14).

CEREBRAL ANGIOGRAPHY PERFORMED WITH COMPUTED TOMOGRAPHY

Elective minimum required is 3.

Common Indications

- Visualization of aneurysms and other vascular pathologic conditions
- Visualization of a subarachnoid or intracranial hemorrhage in the area of the circle of Willis

Imaging Considerations

The basic principle of CT angiography is to acquire information through an area of interest in an adequate amount of time to capture the information in the desired vascular phase. Computed angiography of the intracranial circulation uses a bolus injection of contrast medium, followed by a short delay and spiral scanning only in the area of interest. Spiral imaging has made the visualization of the circle of Willis and other smaller arterial structures during the bolus phase possible. With current 3D imaging, the reconstructed image can be displayed from any imaging plane. Optimal visualization of the vascular area of interest does require precise timing to allow for the maximal flow of contrast medium. The actual time of scanning the area of interest typically does not exceed 60 s.

The area of interest will determine the amount of contrast medium and the delay time. The CT technologist should be familiar with the specific method of determining the delay time for their imaging facility. Certain facilities will determine the specific delay time between injection and image acquisition on each patient. To determine the optimal delay time, the technologist should position the patient in a manner similar to that for a normal brain scan. The prescan image is created from the superior portion of the sella or from the inferior border of the area of interest. The technologist then injects 20 mL of contrast medium in the antecubital vein at a rate of 2.0 mL/s (the injection rate and amount of contrast medium may vary with the standards set by the imaging facility). After the injection of contrast medium, the technologist should wait approximately 8 s and take serial images at the same location. The histogram function is used to determine the peak time of enhancement after the bolus injection.

The actual examination will require the use of approximately 90 mL of contrast medium, a rate of injection of 2.0 mL/s, with a 20-s delay from the onset of contrast injection. The CT angiogram is created by scanning from the inferior to superior border of anatomy. If there is a question of delay time, the technologist should delay slightly longer than the optimal time. If the scan occurs before the peak enhancement phase, there will not be adequate time to rescan and catch the contrast medium before it passes through the area of interest. When demonstrating the circle of Willis, the scan range will include a distance of approximately 5 cm in length. This will allow the visualization of the midbasilar artery and cavernous portions of the carotid arteries to an area superior to the genu of the anterior and middle cerebral arteries. Because the imaging area is restricted to a 5-cm area, the slice thickness should be set for 1 mm when the circle of Willis is the area of interest. The slice thickness should be set at 2 mm when the area of interest is for intracranial circulation. A 1:1 pitch should be used to improve the 3D reconstruction. If a longer scan range is desired, the technologist can increase the pitch to cover the increase in anatomy in the same amount of time. The technologist should remember that both axial and 3D images will be used for their diagnostic values; therefore, the smallest possible slice thickness and lowest pitch will result in an improvement of spatial resolution. To further improve the spatial resolution, the technologist should use a field of view of 12 to 13 cm.

Patient Preparations

The patient is placed supine and head first on the examination table. The head is hyperextended and placed in the head holder. The patient's head is positioned with the midsagittal plane parallel with the longitudinal positioning light. The interpupillary line is parallel with the horizontal positioning light. The technologist should use positioning pads and restraining straps as needed. Place the patient's arms across the abdomen or along the sides. To minimize motion artifacts, the use of restraining straps across the patient's forehead, chin, or both, should be considered. Foam padding placed under the patient's knees can relieve pressure on the lower back and add to the patient's comfort. The patient should be informed to practice quiet breathing and avoid swallowing or other source of unnecessary movement. Thorough but simple instructions involving the imaging procedure will also reduce patient motion. The technologist should remember that the proper placement of radiation shielding is also an essential part of every CT examination.

Imaging Protocols

The first image produced is of the lateral head. From the scout image, the technologist selects the imaging range. The slice thickness is set for 1 mm to accommodate for artifacts created by the petrous pyramids and improve spatial resolution. Angulation of axial slices is often determined by radiologist preference. Certain facilities require the axial slices to be angled parallel with the orbitomeatal line, whereas other facilities prefer an angulation of 15° superior to the orbitomeatal lines. One of the benefits in angulation is the reduction of radiation exposure to the patient's eyes and improved visualization of the posterior fossa.

The images will be reconstructed according to the radiologist preference. There will be approximately 50 axial images completed in the examination. The 3D reconstruction should only include the area of interest and not the area of skull. The use reconstruction algorithms, which eliminate the information from bone and soft tissue, are used in the reconstruction process.

CHAPTER 5

CT Studies of the Neck

The protocol marked with an asterisk must be completed on a patient, not a simulation.

	Mandatory	Elective
Neck		
Larynx		3
Soft tissue*	5*	
Carotid angiography		3

CT EXAMINATION OF THE LARYNX

Elective minimum required is 3.

Common Indications

- Differentiation between soft tissue masses and lymph nodes
- Evaluation of the function of the vocal cords

Imaging Considerations

Imaging of the larynx is typically demonstrated with axial images. The slices within the scan range are normally thin to improve spatial resolution. The axial images should be generated parallel to the vocal cords which also corresponds to the same plane as the cervical disks. Angulation of the slices may be changed to avoid dental artifacts. The FOV should be large enough to include the lateral borders of the neck. Before the examination, the patient should be instructed to avoid swallowing during the imaging process. Some facilities may use a phonation technique for examination of the larynx. During this process, the patient is instructed to pronounce the letter "e" during scanning to evaluate the function of the vocal cords. Imaging of the larynx typically includes the use of intravenous contrast medium to improve the contrast resolution of vascular structures and help identify masses. Contrast medium should be used per facility standards.

The decision to use conventional scanning or spiral scanning is determined by the imaging facility and with consideration to the patient's ability to remain motionless during the examination. An accurate explanation of the examination process with consideration to patient comfort will reduce voluntary motion during the imaging process.

Patient Preparations

AXIAL IMAGES OF THE LARYNX

The patient is placed supine and head first on the examination table. The head is slightly hyperextended and placed in the head holder. The patient's head is positioned with the midsagittal plane parallel with the longitudinal positioning light. The interpupillary line is parallel with the horizontal positioning light. The technologist should use positioning pads and restraining straps as needed. The patient's arms should be placed across the abdomen or along the sides. To minimize motion artifacts, the use of restraining straps across the patient's forehead, chin, or both, should be considered. Foam padding placed under the patient's knees can relieve pressure on the lower back and add to the patient's comfort. Thorough but simple instructions involving the imaging procedure will also reduce patient motion. Proper placement of radiation shielding is also an essential part of every CT examination.

Imaging Protocols

AXIAL IMAGES OF THE LARYNX

The first image produced is the lateral neck. From the scout image, the technologist selects the imaging range from the inferior border of the hyoid bone through the cricoid cartilage. Thin slices are usually selected to improve spatial resolution. The FOV should be large enough to accommodate the lateral borders of the neck. Axial slices are typically angled parallel with the vocal cords, which also corresponds to the cervical disks. To compensate for the angulation, the CT gantry may need to be tilted to the appropriate angle (Fig. 5-1).

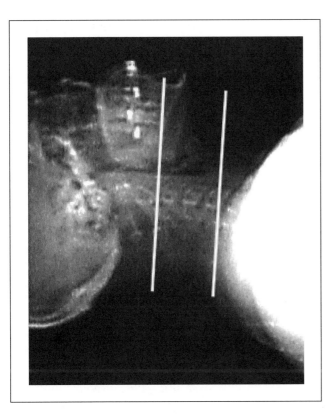

FIGURE 5-1

Lateral view of the larynx with axial slices from the inferior border of the hyoid bone through the cricoid cartilage.

CT EXAMINATION OF THE NECK SOFT TISSUE

Mandatory minimum required is 5. This protocol must be completed on a patient, not a simulation.

Common Indications

- Assessment of soft tissue masses and lymph nodes
- Evaluation of the function of the vocal cords
- Visualization of vascular structures of the neck

Imaging Considerations

Imaging of the neck soft tissue is typically demonstrated with axial images. The slices within the scan range are normally thin to improve spatial resolution. Axial images should be generated parallel to the vocal cords, which also corresponds to the same plane as the cervical disks. Angulation of the slices may be changed to avoid dental artifacts. The FOV should be large enough to include the lateral borders of the neck. Before the examination, the patient should be instructed to avoid swallowing during the imaging process. Some facilities may use a phonation technique for examination of the larynx. During this process, the patient should be instructed to pronounce the letter "e" while scanning to evaluate the function of the vocal cords. Imaging of the neck typically includes the use of intravenous contrast medium to improve the contrast of vascular structures and help identify masses. Contrast medium should be used per facility standards. The decision to use conventional scanning or spiral scanning is determined by the imaging facility and with consideration to the patient's ability to remain motionless during the examination. An accurate explanation of the examination process before the examination and consideration to patient comfort will reduce voluntary motion during the imaging process.

Patient Preparations

AXIAL IMAGES OF THE NECK

The patient is placed supine and head first on the examination table. The head is slightly hyperextended and placed in the head holder. The patient's head is positioned with the midsagittal plane parallel with the longitudinal positioning light. The interpupillary line is parallel with the horizontal positioning light. The technologist should use positioning pads and restraining straps as needed. The patient's arms should be placed across the abdomen or along the sides. To minimize motion artifacts, the use of restraining straps across the patient's forehead, chin, or both, should be considered. Foam padding placed under the patient's knees can relieve pressure on the lower back and add to the patient's comfort. Thorough but simple instructions involving the imaging procedure will also reduce patient motion. Proper placement of radiation shielding is also an essential part of every CT examination.

Imaging Protocols

AXIAL IMAGES OF THE NECK

The first image produced is of the lateral neck. From the scout image, the technologist normally selects the imaging range from the inferior border of the occiput and extends to the first thoracic vertebra. Thin slices are usually selected to improve spatial resolution. The FOV should be large enough to accommodate the lateral borders of the neck. Axial slices are typically angled parallel with the vocal cords, which also corresponds to the cervical disks. To compensate for the angulation, the CT gantry may need to be tilted to the appropriate angle (Fig. 5-2).

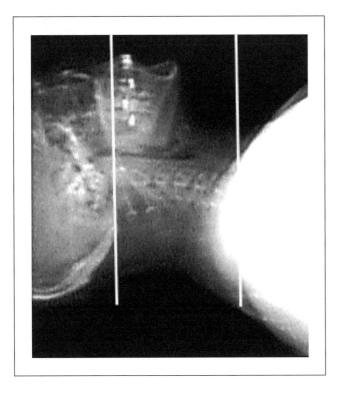

FIGURE 5-2

Lateral view of neck soft tissue with axial slices from the inferior border of the occiput and extends to the first thoracic vertebra.

CAROTID ANGIOGRAPHY

Elective minimum required is 3.

Common Indications

- Suspicion of carotid artery stenosis

Imaging Considerations

The basic principle of CT angiography is to acquire information through an area of interest in an adequate amount of time to capture the information in the desired vascular phase. Computed angiography of the carotid bifurcation uses a bolus injection of contrast medium, followed by a short delay and spiral scanning only in the area of interest. Spiral imaging has made the visualization of carotids and other smaller arterial structures during the bolus phase possible. With current 3D imaging, the reconstructed image can be displayed from any imaging plane. Optimal visualization of the vascular area of interest does require precise timing to allow for the maximal flow of contrast medium. The actual time of scanning the area of interest typically does not exceed 60 s.

The area of interest will determine the amount of contrast medium and the delay time. The CT technologist should be familiar with the specific method of determining the delay time for their imaging facility. Certain facilities will determine the specific delay time between injection and image acquisition on each patient. To determine the optimal delay time, the technologist should position the patient in a manner similar to that for a normal neck scan. Most carotids will bifurcate in the area of C6-7; for this reason, the examination table is positioned at this location for the prescan image. The technologist then injects 20 mL of contrast medium in the antecubital vein at a rate of 2.0 mL/s (the injection rate and amount of contrast medium may vary with the standards set by the imaging facility). After injection of contrast medium, the technologist should wait approximately 8 s and take serial images with 1- to 2-s intervals at the same location. The histogram function is used to determine the peak time of enhancement after the bolus injection.

The actual examination will require the use of approximately 75 mL of contrast medium at a rate of injection of 2.0 mL/s, with approximately 25-s delay from the onset of the contrast injection. The CT angiogram is created by scanning from the inferior to superior border of anatomy. If a there is a question of delay time, the technologist should delay slightly longer than the optimal time. If the scan occurs before the peak enhancement phase, there will not be adequate time to rescan and catch the contrast medium before it passes through the area of interest. The scan should start at the base of the neck and proceed superior for approximately 18 cm. This will ensure that the complete region of the bifurcation can be imaged in 60 s or less. Because the imaging area is restricted to a 18-cm area, the slice thickness should be set for 3 mm to scan through the area of interest in a single scan range. A 1:1 pitch should be used to improve the 3D reconstruction. If a longer scan range is desired, the technologist can increase the pitch to cover the increase in anatomy in the same amount of time. The technologist should remember that both axial and 3D images will be used for their diagnostic values; therefore, the smallest possible slice thickness and lowest pitch will result in an improvement of spatial resolution. To further improve the spatial resolution, the technologist should use an FOV to cover only the area of interest.

Patient Preparations

The patient is placed supine and head first on the examination table. The head is hyperextended and placed in the head holder. The patient's neck is positioned with the midsagittal plane parallel with the longitudinal positioning light. The interpupillary line is parallel with the horizontal positioning light. The technologist should use positioning pads and restraining straps as needed. Place the patient's arms across the abdomen or along the sides. To minimize motion artifacts, the use of restraining straps across the patient's forehead, chin, or both, should be considered. Foam padding placed under the patient's knees can relieve pressure on the lower back and add to the patient's comfort. The patient should be informed to practice quiet breathing and avoid swallowing or other sources of unnecessary movement. Thorough but simple instructions involving the imaging procedure will also reduce patient motion. The technologist should remember that the proper placement of radiation shielding is also an essential part of every CT examination.

Imaging Protocols

The first image produced is of the lateral neck. From the scout image, the technologist selects the imaging range, starting at the base of the neck or T1. The slice thickness is set for 3 mm to accommodate for the distance of the scan range and improve spatial resolution. There is no angulation of axial slices. There will be approximately 60 axial images completed in the examination. The images will be reconstructed according to the radiologist preference. The 3D reconstruction should only include the area of interest and not the area of upper skull or chest. The use reconstruction algorithms, which eliminate the information from bone and soft tissue, are used in the reconstruction process.

CHAPTER 6

CT Imaging Procedures of the Spine

The protocol marked with an asterisk must be completed on a patient, not a simulation.

	Mandatory	Elective
Spine		
Cervical	5	
Thoracic		3
Lumbosacral*	5*	
Postmyelography	3	

CT EXAMINATION OF THE CERVICAL SPINE

Mandatory minimum required is 5.

Common Indications

- Evaluation of herniated disk or trauma
- Evaluation of degenerative disk disease
- Detection of neoplasm or infection
- Evaluation of spinal infection
- Evaluation of spinal stenosis

Imaging Considerations

Imaging of the cervical spine is typically demonstrated with axial images. The slices within the scan range are normally thin to improve spatial resolution. The axial images should be parallel to the majority of the cervical disks. The FOV should be large enough to include the lateral borders of the neck. Before the examination, the patient should be instructed to avoid swallowing during the imaging process. Typically, imaging of the cervical spine does not use intravenous contrast medium except when trying to help identify masses. Contrast medium should be used per facility standards. The decision to use conventional scanning or spiral scanning is determined by the imaging facility and with consideration to the patient's ability to remain motionless during the examination. An accurate explanation of the examination process before the examination and consideration to patient comfort will reduce voluntary motion during the imaging process.

Patient Preparations

AXIAL IMAGES OF THE CERVICAL SPINE

The patient is placed supine and head first on the examination table. The head is slightly hyperextended and placed in the head holder. Position the patient's head with the midsagittal plane parallel with the longitudinal positioning light. The interpupillary line is parallel with the horizontal positioning light. The technologist should use positioning pads and restraining straps as needed. The technologist should have the patient relax the shoulders in a comfortable position. The patient's arms should be placed across the abdomen or along the sides. To minimize motion artifacts, the use of restraining straps across the patient's forehead, chin, or both, should be considered. Foam padding placed under the patient's knees can relieve pressure on the lower back and add to the patient's comfort, which reduces the likelihood of patient motion. Thorough but simple instructions involving the imaging procedure will also reduce patient motion. Proper placement of radiation shielding is also an essential part of every CT examination.

Imaging Protocols

AXIAL IMAGES OF THE CERVICAL SPINE

The first image produced is an anterior to posterior view of the neck. From the scout image, the technologist normally determines whether

FIGURE 6-1

Anteroposterior view of the cervical spine to show proper centering and alignment.

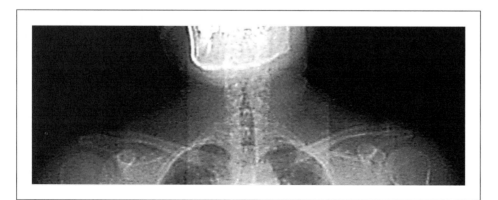

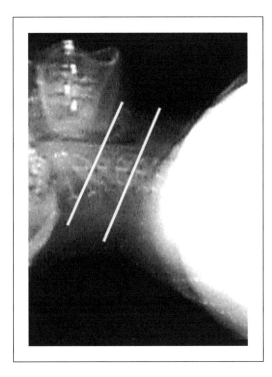

FIGURE 6-2

Lateral view of the cervical spine with axial slices angled parallel with the cervical disks.

the midsagittal plane of the patient is centered to the long axis of the examination table. The technologist should also select a lateral scout of the cervical spine to determine the range of axial slices. The axial slices should be parallel with the angle of the cervical disks. The typical cervical spine is not examined to its full length. Normally the technologist, radiologist, or both, will select specific areas within the spine to be examined. This should only be through one or two disks. Thin slices are usually selected to improve spatial resolution. To compensate for the angulation, the CT gantry may need to be tilted to the appropriate angle (Figs. 6-1 and 6-2).

CT EXAMINATION OF THE THORACIC SPINE

Elective minimum required is 3.

Common Indications

- Evaluation of herniated disk or trauma
- Evaluation of degenerative disk disease
- Detection of neoplasm or infection
- Evaluation of spinal infection
- Evaluation of spinal stenosis

Imaging Considerations

Imaging of the thoracic spine is typically demonstrated with axial images. The slices within the scan range are normally thin to improve spatial resolution. The axial images should be parallel to the majority of the thoracic disks. The FOV should be large enough to include the anterior border of the aorta and the posterior spinous process. Imaging of the thoracic spine typically does not use intravenous contrast medium except when trying to help identify masses. Contrast medium should be used per facility standards. The decision to use conventional scanning or spiral scanning is determined by the imaging facility and with consideration to the patient's ability to remain motionless during the examination. An accurate explanation of the examination process before the examination and consideration to patient comfort will reduce voluntary motion during the imaging process.

Patient Preparations

AXIAL IMAGES OF THE THORACIC SPINE

The patient is placed supine and head first on the examination table. The patient's body should be aligned so the midsagittal plane is centered to the examination table. The horizontal positioning light should pass though the center of the thoracic spine. The technologist

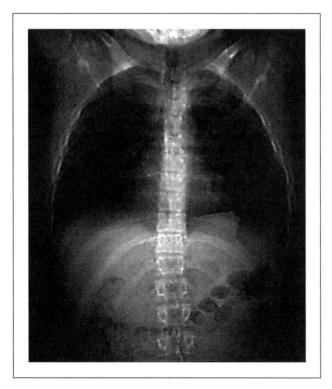

FIGURE 6-3

Anteroposterior view of the thoracic spine to show proper centering and alignment.

should use positioning pads and restraining straps as needed. The patient's arms should be placed above the head when scanning the thoracic spine. Foam padding placed under the patient's knees can relieve pressure on the lower back and add to the patient's comfort. Thorough but simple instructions involving the imaging procedure will also reduce patient motion. The proper placement of radiation shielding is also an essential part of every CT examination.

Imaging Protocols

AXIAL IMAGES OF THE THORACIC SPINE

The first image produced is an anterior to posterior view of the thoracic spine. From the scout image, the technologist normally determines whether the midsagittal plane of the patient is centered to the long axis of the examination table. The technologist should also select a lateral scout of the thoracic spine to determine the range of axial slices. The axial slices should be parallel with the angle of the thoracic disks. The typical thoracic spine is not examined to its full length. Normally, the technologist, radiologist, or both, will select specific areas within the spine to be examined. This should only be through one or two disks. The technologist should select the ranges accordingly. These ranges are normally from the pedicle superior to the area of interest through the pedicle inferior to the area of interest. To compensate for the angulation, the CT gantry may need to be tilted to the appropriate angle. Thin slices are usually selected to improve spatial resolution. The FOV of the axial images should include the anterior border of the aorta and the posterior spinous process (Figs. 6-3 and 6-4).

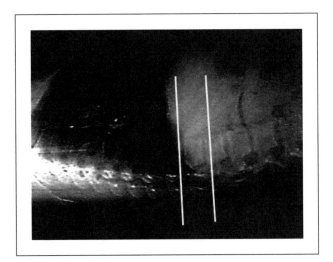

FIGURE 6-4

Lateral view of the thoracic spine with axial slices angled parallel with the thoracic disks.

CT EXAMINATION OF THE LUMBOSACRAL SPINE

Mandatory minimum required is 5. This protocol must be completed on a patient, not a simulation.

Common Indications

- Evaluation of herniated disk or trauma
- Evaluation of degenerative disk disease
- Detection of neoplasm or infection
- Evaluation of spinal infection
- Evaluation of spinal stenosis

Imaging Considerations

Imaging of the lumbosacral spine is typically demonstrated with axial images. The slices within the scan range are normally thin to improve spatial resolution. The axial images should be parallel to the lumbar disks. The FOV should be large enough to include the anterior border of the aorta and the posterior spinous process. Imaging of the lumbosacral spine typically does not use intravenous contrast medium except when trying to help identify masses or to differentiate scar tissue from recurrent disk disease in the postsurgical spine. Contrast medium should be used per facility standards. The decision to use conventional scanning or spiral scanning is determined by the imaging facility and with consideration to the patient's ability to remain motionless during the examination. An accurate explanation of the examination process before the examination and consideration to patient comfort will reduce voluntary motion during the imaging process.

Patient Preparations

AXIAL IMAGES OF THE LUMBOSACRAL SPINE

The patient is placed supine and head first on the examination table. The patient's body should be aligned so that the midsagittal plane is centered to the examination table. The horizontal positioning light should pass though the center of the lumbar spine. The technologist should use positioning pads and restraining straps as needed. The patient's arms should be placed above the head or across the chest when scanning the lumbar spine. Foam padding placed under the patient's knees can reduce the natural lordotic curvature of the lumbar spine and add to the patient's comfort, which will reduce the likelihood of patient motion. Thorough but simple instructions involving the imaging procedure will also reduce patient motion. The proper placement of radiation shielding is also an essential part of every CT examination.

Imaging Protocols

AXIAL IMAGES OF THE LUMBOSACRAL SPINE

The first image produced is an anterior to posterior view of the lumbosacral spine. From the scout image, the technologist normally determines whether the midsagittal plane of the patient is centered to the long axis of the examination table. The technologist should also select a lateral scout of the lumbosacral spine to determine the range of axial slices. The axial slices should be parallel with the angle of the lumbar disks. The typical lumbosacral spine is not examined to its full length. Normally the technologist, radiologist, or both, will select specific areas within the spine to be examined. This should only be through three or four disks. These ranges are normally from the pedicle superior to the area of interest through the pedicle inferior to the area of interest. To compensate for the angulation, the CT gantry may need to be tilted to the appropriate angle. Thin slices are usually selected to improve spatial resolution. The FOV of the axial images should include the transverse and posterior spinous process and associated muscles (Figs. 6-5 and 6-6).

FIGURE 6-5

Anteroposterior view of the lumbar spine to show proper centering and alignment.

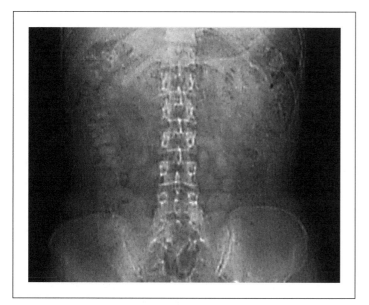

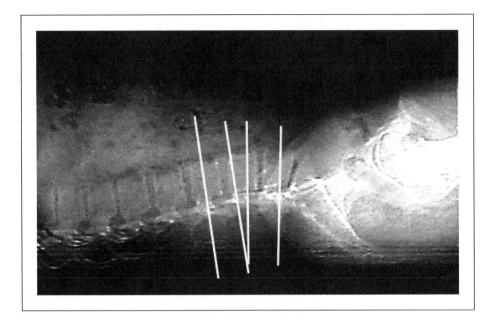

FIGURE 6-6

Lateral view of the lumbar spine with axial slices angled parallel with the lumbar disks.

CT EXAMINATION OF THE POSTMYELOGRAPHIC SPINE

Mandatory minimum required is 3.

Common Indications

• Clarification of intradural and extradural abnormalities

Imaging Considerations

Imaging of the postmyelographic spine is typically demonstrated with axial images. The examination is similar to that of a normal CT spine examination. The intrathecal contrast medium is present from the previous radiographic procedure. The CT postmyelographic examination is typically completed within 1 to 4 h of the administration of intrathecal contrast medium. The delay time is to allow the contrast medium adequate time to dilute, because dense contrast medium may obscure intradural structures. Some facilities will have the patient completely roll over to prevent layering of the cerebral spinal fluid and the contrast medium. The patient should also be positioned with the head slightly elevated to avoid headaches and seizures.

The slices within the scan range are normally thin to improve spatial resolution. The axial images should be parallel to the disks. The FOV should be large enough to include the anterior border of the vertebral body and the spinous process. The decision to use conventional scanning or spiral scanning is determined by the imaging facility and with consideration to the patient's ability to remain motionless during the examination. An accurate explanation of the examination process before the examination and consideration to patient comfort will reduce voluntary motion during the imaging process.

Patient Preparations

AXIAL IMAGES OF THE POSTMYELOGRAPHIC SPINE

The patient is placed supine and head first on the examination table. The patient's head should be slightly elevated to prevent headaches or seizures. The patient's body should be aligned so that the midsagittal plane is centered to the examination table. The horizontal positioning light should pass though the center of the spine. The technologist should use positioning pads and restraining straps as needed. The patient should place the arms out of the area to be scanned. To minimize motion artifacts, the use of restraining straps should be considered. Foam padding placed under the patient's knees can reduce the natural lordotic curvature of the lumbar spine and add to the patient's comfort. Thorough but simple instructions involving the imaging procedure will also reduce patient motion. The proper placement of radiation shielding is also an essential part of every CT examination.

Imaging Protocols

AXIAL IMAGES OF THE POSTMYELOGRAPHIC SPINE

The first image produced is an anterior to posterior view of the spine. From the scout image, the technologist normally determines whether the midsagittal plane of the patient is centered to the long axis of the examination table. The technologist should also select a lateral scout of the spine to determine the range of axial slices. The axial slices should be parallel with the angle of the disks. The typical postmyelographic spine is examined only in the area of interest. Normally, the technologist, radiologist, or both, will select specific areas within the spine to be examined. To compensate for the angulation, the CT gantry may need to be tilted to the appropriate angle. Thin slices are usually selected to improve spatial resolution. The FOV of the axial images should include the transverse and posterior spinous process.

CHAPTER 7

CT Imaging Procedures of the Chest

The protocol marked with an asterisk must be completed on a patient, not a simulation.

	Mandatory
Chest	
Mediastinum*	10*
Vascular	5 (including heart and great vessels)
Lung	5
High-resolution computed tomography	5

CT EXAMINATION OF THE MEDIASTINUM

Mandatory minimum required is 10. This procedure must be completed on a patient not a simulation.

Common Indications

- Visualization of pulmonary masses
- Demonstration of hilar lymph nodes and masses
- Demonstration of aortic aneurysms

Imaging Considerations

Imaging of the mediastinum is typically demonstrated with axial images. The axial images of the mediastinum require no angulation of the gantry. Intravenous contrast medium can be used to demonstrate hilar masses, lymphoma, and cardiac masses as well as enhancing the aorta and other vessels of the chest. Contrast medium should be used according to facility standards. The FOV is set large enough to include the lateral borders of the chest. Before the examination, the patient should be instructed on proper breathing technique. The decision to use conventional scanning or spiral scanning is determined by the imaging facility and with consideration to the patient's ability to remain motionless during the examination. An accurate explanation of the examination process and consideration to patient comfort will reduce voluntary motion during the imaging process.

Patient Preparations

AXIAL IMAGES OF THE MEDIASTINUM

The patient is placed supine and head first on the examination table. Position the patient with the midsagittal plane of the patient parallel with the longitudinal positioning light. The technologist should use positioning pads and restraining straps as needed. The patient's arms should be above the head. To minimize motion artifacts, the use of restraining straps should be considered. Foam padding placed under the patient's knees can relieve pressure on the lower back and add to the patient's comfort, which reduces the likelihood of patient motion. The patient should be informed of proper breathing techniques before the start of the examination. Thorough but simple instructions involving the imaging procedure will also reduce patient motion. The proper placement of radiation shielding is also an essential part of every CT examination.

Imaging Protocols

AXIAL IMAGES OF THE MEDIASTINUM

The first image produced is a coronal view of the chest. From the scout image, the technologist normally determines whether the mid-

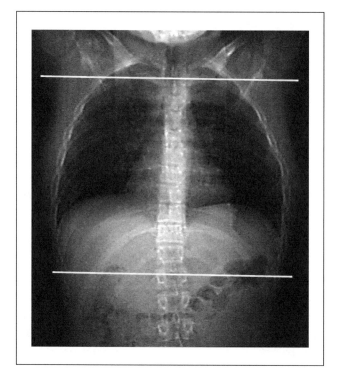

FIGURE 7-1

Coronal view of the chest with axial slices extending from the sternal notch through the level of the adrenal glands.

sagittal plane of the patient is centered relative to the long axis of the examination table. The range of axial images should extend from the sternal notch through the level of the adrenal glands. Some facilities will use a range of 5-mm slices through the area of the mediastinum and 10-mm slices once through the mediastinum. The thin slices will reduce volume imaging and improve spatial resolution. The technologist should select a large FOV to accommodate the entire chest. The axial slices should be perpendicular to the midsagittal plane of the patient (Fig. 7-1).

CT EXAMINATION OF THE VASCULAR STRUCTURES OF THE HEART AND GREAT VESSELS

Mandatory minimum required is 5.

Common Indications

- Differentiation of mediastinal pathologic conditions such as lymphadenopathy and solid masses from fatty and cystic lesions
- Evaluation of anomalies, aneurysms, dissections, and coarctation

Imaging Considerations

The basic principle of CT angiography is to acquire information through an area of interest in an adequate amount of time to capture the information in the desired vascular phase. Computed angiography of the heart and great vessels uses a bolus injection of contrast medium, followed by a short delay and spiral scanning only in the area of interest. Spiral imaging has made the visualization of vascular structures during the bolus phase possible. With current 3D imaging, the reconstructed image can be displayed from any imaging plane. Optimal visualization of the vascular area of interest does require precise timing to allow for the maximal flow of contrast medium. The actual time of scanning the area of interest typically does not exceed 60 s.

The area of interest will determine the amounts and delay times of contrast medium. The CT technologist should be familiar with the specific method of determining the delay time for the imaging facility. Certain facilities will determine the specific delay time between injection and image acquisition on each patient. To determine the optimal delay time, the technologist should position the patient in a manner similar to that for a normal chest scan. Position the examination table at the area of interest for the prescan image. The technologist then injects 20 mL of contrast medium in the antecubital vein at a rate of 2.0 mL/s (the injection rate and amount of contrast medium may vary with the standards set by the imaging facility). After the injection of contrast medium, the technologist should wait approximately 8 s and take serial images with 1- to 2-s intervals at the same location. The histogram function is used to determine the peak time of enhancement after the bolus injection.

The actual examination will require the use of approximately 60 mL of contrast medium at a rate of injection of 2.0 mL/s. The CT angiogram is created by scanning from the superior to inferior borders of the area of interest. If there is a question of delay time, the technologist should delay slightly longer than the optimal time. If the scan occurs before the peak enhancement phase, there will not be adequate time to rescan and catch the contrast medium before it passes through the area of interest. The technologist should remember that both axial and 3D images will be used for the diagnostic values; therefore, the smallest possible slice thickness and lowest pitch will result in an improvement of spatial resolution. The combination should still accommodate the entire area of interest in a single scan range. If a longer scan range is desired, the technologist can increase the pitch to cover the increase in anatomy in the same amount of time. To further improve the spatial resolution, the technologist should use an FOV to cover only the area of interest.

Patient Preparations

The patient is placed supine and head first on the examination table. The patient's chest is positioned with the midsagittal plane of the patient parallel with the longitudinal positioning light. The table height should allow the horizontal positioning light to intersect the midcoronal plane of the patient. The technologist should use positioning pads and restraining straps as needed. Place the patient's arms above the head. To minimize motion artifacts, the use of restraining straps should be considered. Foam padding placed under the patient's knees can relieve pressure on the lower back and add to the patient's comfort. The patient should be instructed on proper breath-holding techniques. Thorough but simple instructions involving the imaging procedure will also reduce patient motion. The technologist should remember that the proper placement of radiation shielding is also an essential part of every CT examination.

Imaging Protocols

The first image produced is a coronal view of the chest. From the scout image, the technologist selects the imaging range starting at the superior border of the mediastinum. The slice thickness is set to accommodate for the distance of the scan range and improve spatial resolution. There is no angulation of axial slices. The images will be reconstructed according to the radiologist preference. The 3D reconstruction should only include the area of interest and not the entire chest. The use reconstruction algorithms, which eliminate the information from bone and soft tissue, are used in the reconstruction process.

CT EXAMINATION OF THE LUNGS

Mandatory minimum required is 5.

Common Indications

- Differentiating lung nodules from pulmonary blood vessels
- Detection of pulmonary metastases
- Definition of pleural effusions
- Evaluation of aortic aneurysms
- Evaluation of thoracic abscesses

Imaging Considerations

Lung imaging is typically demonstrated with axial images. The axial images require no angulation of the gantry. Intravenous contrast medium can be used to differentiate masses from mediastinal vessels. Contrast medium is also helpful in assessment of vascular malformations. Contrast medium should be used per facility standards. The FOV should be large enough to include the lateral borders of the chest. Before the examination, the patient should be instructed on proper breathing techniques. The decision to use conventional scanning or spiral scanning is determined by the imaging facility and with consideration to the patient's ability to remain motionless during the examination. An accurate explanation of the examination process before the examination and consideration to patient comfort will reduce voluntary motion during the imaging process.

Patient Preparations

AXIAL IMAGES OF THE LUNGS

The patient is placed supine and head first on the examination table. The patient is positioned with the midsagittal plane of the patient parallel with the longitudinal positioning light. The technologist should use positioning pads and restraining straps as needed. The patient's arms should be above the head. To minimize motion artifacts, the use of restraining straps should be considered. Foam padding placed under the patient's knees can relieve pressure on the lower back and add to the patient's comfort, which reduces the likelihood of patient motion. The patient should be informed of proper breathing techniques before the start of the examination. Thorough but simple instructions involving the imaging procedure will also reduce patient motion. The proper placement of radiation shielding is also an essential part of every CT examination.

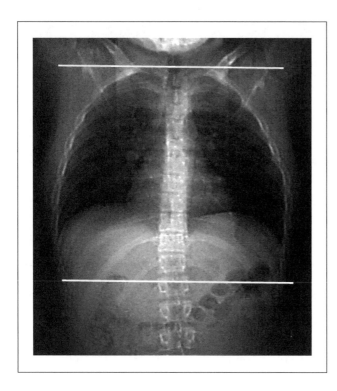

FIGURE 7-2
Coronal view of the chest with axial slices extending from the sternal notch or apex of the lungs through the level of the adrenal glands.

Imaging Protocols

AXIAL IMAGES OF THE LUNGS

The first image produced is a coronal view of the chest. From the scout image, the technologist normally determines whether the midsagittal plane of the patient is centered relative to the long axis of the examination table. The range of axial images should extend from the sternal notch or apex of the lungs through the level of the adrenal glands. Some facilities will use a range of 5-mm slices through the area of the mediastinum and 10-mm slices once through the mediastinum. The thin slices will reduce volume imaging and improve spatial resolution. The technologist should select a large FOV to accommodate the entire chest. The axial slices should be perpendicular to the midsagittal plane of the patient (Fig. 7-2).

HIGH-RESOLUTION CT EXAMINATION OF THE LUNGS

Mandatory minimum required is 5.

Common Indications

- Evaluation of the lungs for interstitial disease or subtle air space consolidation
- Evaluation of fine lung structures and airways
- Evaluation of patients for emphysema and asbestosis

Imaging Considerations

The purpose of high-resolution CT examinations is to optimize the spatial resolution of the scanner. For specific areas within the lungs, the technologist should consider the use of thin slices, such as 1 to 2 mm. When the entire lungs are to be demonstrated, the choice of 8- to 10-mm slices should be considered. In either case, the technologist should select a high spatial-frequency reconstruction algorithm. Departments vary in the imaging protocol for high-resolution studies. Some departments will only use high-resolution imaging in the area of interest as well as the one slice at the apex, hilar area, and base of the lung. The technologist should have a firm understanding of the departmental protocol involving high-resolution CT imaging before the examination.

Typically, high-resolution lung imaging is demonstrated with axial images. The axial images require no angulation of the gantry. Intravenous contrast medium can be used to differentiate masses from mediastinal vessels. Contrast medium is also helpful in assessment of vascular malformations. Contrast medium should be used per facility standards. The FOV should be large enough to include the lateral borders of the chest. Before the examination, the patient should be instructed on proper breathing techniques. The decision to use conventional scanning or spiral scanning is determined by the imaging facility and with consideration to the patient's ability to remain motionless during the examination. An accurate explanation of the examination process before the examination and consideration to patient comfort will reduce voluntary motion during the imaging process.

Patient Preparations

AXIAL IMAGES FOR HIGH-RESOLUTION SCAN OF LUNGS

The patient is placed supine and head first on the examination table. The patient is positioned with the midsagittal plane of the patient parallel with the longitudinal positioning lights. Use positioning pads and restraining straps as needed. The patient's arms should be above the head. To minimize motion artifacts, the use of restraining straps should be considered. Foam padding placed under the patient's knees can relieve pressure on the lower back and add to the patient's comfort, which reduces the likelihood of patient motion. The patient should be informed of proper breathing techniques before the start of the examination. Thorough but simple instructions involving the imaging procedure will also reduce patient motion. The proper placement of radiation shielding is also an essential part of every CT examination.

Imaging Protocols

AXIAL IMAGES FOR HIGH-RESOLUTION SCAN OF LUNGS

The first image produced is a coronal view of the chest. From the scout image, the technologist normally determines whether the midsagittal plane of the patient is centered relative to the long axis of the examination table. The range of axial images should extend from the sternal notch or apex of the lungs and extend through the level of the adrenal glands. Some facilities will use a range of 5-mm slices through the area of the mediastinum and 10-mm slices once through the mediastinum. The thin slices will reduce volume imaging and improve spatial resolution. The technologist should select a large FOV to accommodate the entire chest. The axial slices should be perpendicular to the midsagittal plane of the patient.

CHAPTER 8

CT Imaging Procedures of the Abdomen and Pelvis

The protocol marked with an asterisk must be completed on a patient, not a simulation.

Abdomen and pelvis	Mandatory	Elective
Routine abdomen*	10*	
Liver	5	
GI tract		3
Pancreas	5	
Adrenals		3
Kidneys	5	
Vascular abdomen	5	
Routine pelvis	5	

CT EXAMINATION OF THE ABDOMEN

Mandatory minimum required is 10. This procedure must be completed on a patient, not a simulation.

Common Indications

- Detection of abdominal masses and lesions
- Detection of vascular abnormalities of liver, spleen, kidneys, and gastrointestinal tract

Imaging Considerations

PRE-EXAMINATION PREPARATION

Preparation for the abdominal CT examination may vary slightly for each imaging center or radiologist preference. The CT technologist must be aware of the specific protocol before scheduling the patient for an examination. Preparation of abdominal scanning typically begins the night before the actual imaging process. When the scan is to be completed the following morning, the patient will usually have a clear liquid supper the night before the examination and have nothing by mouth (NPO) after midnight. If the CT scan is scheduled for the afternoon, the patient will consume a clear liquid supper and breakfast the day of the afternoon scan. The patient will be NPO after breakfast on the day of the afternoon scan. In either case of a morning or afternoon CT examination, the patient typically takes a laxative the evening before the scan. It is important that the patient understands that the presence of fecal matter can appear as a pathologic mass within the alimentary tract and restrict the flow of oral contrast medium.

ORAL CONTRAST ENHANCEMENT

Imaging of the abdomen normally uses a combination of oral and intravenous contrast media. Oral contrast medium will differentiate the loops of bowel from a mass or an abnormal fluid collection. Two commonly used oral contrast agents are barium sulfate or water soluble based. The area of interest will determine the amount and time the contrast medium should be consumed. For example, when scanning the upper abdomen the patient should consume approximately 400 mL of oral contrast medium 15 to 30 min in advance of the scanning. At the time of the scan, the patient will drink another 300 mL of contrast medium. For visualization of the lower abdomen and pelvis, the patient will consume 1200 mL of oral contrast medium 30 to 45 min prior to the scan, and another 300 mL of contrast is taken at the time of the scan. The purpose of the last 300 mL of contrast agent is to opacify the duodenum. The imaging facility and radiologist will dictate the type and timing for oral contrast medium.

INTRAVENOUS CONTRAST ENHANCEMENT

Intravenous contrast medium is used to enhance vascular structures such as the portal vein, abdominal aorta, inferior vena cava, and iliac arteries and veins. In addition, intravenous contrast medium is used for the visualization of the ureters and bladder. Imaging of the abdomen normally requires the use of intravenous contrast medium. When using intravenous contrast medium, it is left to the discretion of the imaging facility to determine the optimal injection rates and amounts of contrast to be used. It is the responsibility of the technologist to be familiar with all contraindications for the use of intravenous contrast medium. With vascular imaging of the abdomen, some facilities use a single bolus injection followed by a delay before imaging. Other facilities may use multiple bolus injections with different flow rates. The technologist should be aware of the facility standards before using intravenous contrast.

There is controversy as to whether to perform an abdomen study with and without intravenous contrast medium or to perform a study with intravenous contrast alone. In cases for which there is a dual study, the noncontrast portion is completed first. The imaging of the noncontrast abdomen ranges from the xiphoid tip and extends to the iliac crest. If the pelvis is to be scanned as part of the abdomen study, the pelvis will be scanned during the second part of the study and will follow the contrast injection. The second portion of the study will resume scanning at the xiphoid tip and continue through the symphysis pubis. When using intravenous contrast medium, it is important to determine the area of interest. This will designate the rate of contrast injection and the postinjection delay before the technologist starts to scan. The technologist should be aware of the facility standards when considering the imaging protocol.

Patient Preparations

The patient is placed supine and head first on the examination table with the midsagittal plane of the patient parallel with the longitudinal positioning lights. The midcoronal plane of the patient should pass through the center of the horizontal plane of the CT gantry. The patient's arms should be above the head. To minimize motion artifacts, the use of positioning pads and restraining straps should be considered. Foam padding placed under the patient's knees can relieve pressure on the lower back and add to the patient's comfort, which reduces the likelihood of patient motion. The patient should be informed of proper breathing techniques before the start of the examination. Thorough but simple instructions involving the imaging procedure will also reduce patient motion. The decision to use conventional scanning or spiral scanning is determined by the imaging facility, with consideration to the patient's ability to remain motionless during the examination. The proper placement of radiation shielding is also an essential part of every CT examination.

Imaging Protocols

NONINTRAVENOUS CONTRAST STUDY OF THE ABDOMEN

The first image produced is a coronal view of the abdomen. From the scout image, the technologist normally determines whether the midsagittal plane of the patient is centered relative to the long axis of the examination table. The range of axial images should extend from the xiphoid tip through the level of the iliac crest. The technologist should select a large FOV to accommodate the entire abdomen. The axial slices should be perpendicular to the midsagittal plane of the patient and do not require angulation of the gantry (Fig. 8-1).

69

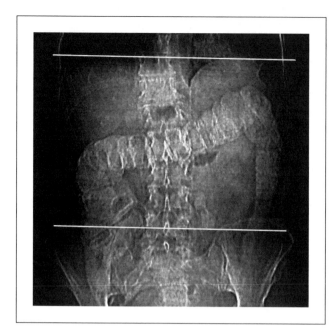

FIGURE 8-1

Coronal view of the abdomen with axial slices extending from the xiphoid tip through the level of the iliac crest.

INTRAVENOUS CONTRAST STUDY OF THE ABDOMEN

Upon completion of the nonintravenous contrast study, the technologist repositions the patient at the location of the xiphoid tip. After the injection and appropriate delay of intravenous contrast medium, the second part of the scanning procedure begins. The second scanning procedure typically goes from the xiphoid tip through the symphysis. The CT scanner may require a delay following the range from the xiphoid tip to the adrenal glands. This delay will allow for the contrast medium to reach the patient's kidneys. After a second delay, the technologist can complete the study by scanning the range from the adrenal glands through the bladder. The selection of delay times and separate scan ranges is dependent on the imaging facility (Fig. 8-2).

CT IMAGING OF THE LIVER

Mandatory minimum required is 5.

Common Indications

- Evaluation of liver abnormalities such as fatty infiltration, cirrhosis, hemochromatosis, hematoma, abscesses, lymphoma, and metastases

70

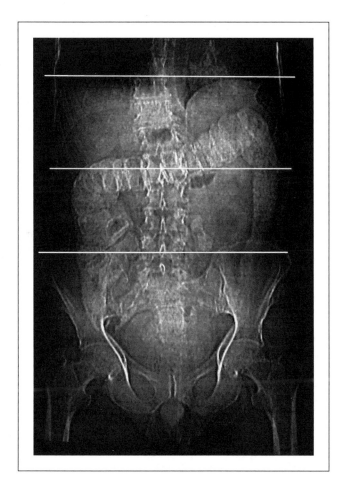

FIGURE 8-2

Coronal view (contrast study) of the abdomen with axial slices extending from the xiphoid tip to the adrenals. The second range is from the adrenals through the level of the iliac crest.

Imaging Considerations

PRE-EXAMINATION PREPARATION

Preparation for the CT examination of the liver may vary slightly for each imaging center or radiologist preference. The CT technologist must be aware of the specific protocol before scheduling the patient for an examination. Preparation of abdominal scanning typically begins the night before the actual imaging process. When the scan is to be completed the following morning, the patient will usually have a clear liquid supper the night before the examination and have NPO after midnight. If the CT scan is scheduled for the afternoon, the patient will consume a clear liquid supper and breakfast the day of the afternoon scan. The patient will be NPO after breakfast on the day of the afternoon scan. In either case of a morning or afternoon CT examination, the patient typically takes a laxative the evening before the scan. It is important that the patient understands that the presence of fecal matter can appear as a pathologic mass within the alimentary tract and restrict the flow of oral contrast medium.

71

ORAL CONTRAST ENHANCEMENT

Imaging of the liver normally is performed using a combination of oral and intravenous contrast media. Oral contrast medium will differentiate the loops of bowel from a mass or an abnormal fluid collection. Two commonly used oral contrast agents are barium sulfate or water soluble based. The area of interest will determine the amount and time the contrast medium should be consumed. The imaging facility and radiologist will dictate the type and timing for oral contrast medium.

INTRAVENOUS CONTRAST ENHANCEMENT

Intravenous contrast medium is used to enhance vascular structures such as the portal veins, hepatic veins, abdominal aorta, and inferior vena cava. Imaging of the liver normally requires the use of intravenous contrast medium. When using intravenous contrast medium, it is left to the discretion of the imaging facility to determine the optimal injection rates and amounts of contrast to be used. It is the responsibility of the technologist to be familiar with all contraindications for the use of intravenous contrast medium. For vascular imaging of the liver, some facilities use a single bolus injection followed by a delay before imaging. Other facilities may use multiple bolus injections with different flow rates. When using intravenous contrast medium, it is important to determine the area of interest. This determination will designate the rate of contrast injection and the postinjection delay before the technologist starts to scan. The technologist should be aware of the facility standards when considering the imaging protocol.

Patient Preparations

The patient is placed supine and head first on the examination table with the midsagittal plane of the patient parallel with the longitudinal positioning lights. The midcoronal plane of the patient should pass through the center of the horizontal plane of the CT gantry. The patient's arms should be above the head. To minimize motion artifacts, the use of positioning pads and restraining straps should be considered. Foam padding placed under the patient's knees can relieve pressure on the lower back and add to the patient's comfort, which reduces the likelihood of patient motion. The patient should be informed of proper breathing techniques before the start of the examination. Thorough but simple instructions involving the imaging procedure will also reduce patient motion. The decision to use conventional scanning or spiral scanning is determined by the imaging facility, with consideration to the patient's ability to remain motionless during the examination. The proper placement of radiation shielding is also an essential part of every CT examination.

Imaging Protocols

Imaging of the liver is not routinely completed as an individual examination. A routine CT examination of the abdomen and pelvis, with attention to the liver, is more of a typical examination process. The technologist may consider a thinner slice thickness to improve image quality when scanning the area of interest.

NONINTRAVENOUS CONTRAST STUDY WITH AXIAL IMAGES OF THE LIVER

The first image produced is a coronal view of the abdomen. From the scout image, the technologist determines whether the midsagittal plane of the patient is centered relative to the long axis of the examination table. The range of axial images should extend from the dome of the liver through the inferior border of the right lobe. The technologist selects a large FOV to accommodate the entire abdomen. The axial slices require no angulation of the gantry and should be perpendicular to the midsagittal plane of the patient (Fig. 8-3).

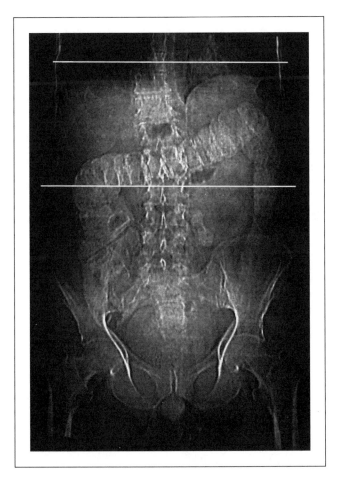

FIGURE 8-3

Coronal view of the liver with axial slices extending from the dome of the liver through the inferior border of the right lobe.

INTRAVENOUS CONTRAST STUDY WITH AXIAL IMAGES OF THE LIVER

Upon completion of the nonintravenous contrast study, the technologist repositions the patient at the beginning location of the xiphoid tip. Contrast injections for studies of the liver are critical. Optimal differentiation between healthy liver tissue and abnormalities occurs during the nonequilibrium phase. During the equilibrium phase, the tumors enhance with presence of contrast medium and, therefore, give the liver an isodense appearance. When using conventional CT scanning of the liver, many facilities inject 100 to 150 mL of iodinated contrast at the rate of 1.5 to 2.0 mL/s. The remainder of the intravenous contrast is injected at 1 mL/s. The second injection will continue to enhance the vasculature of the abdomen.

If spiral scanning is the choice for abdominal imaging, the injection rate of 1.5 to 2.0 mL/s is used for the entire amount of contrast medium. This rate will accommodate for the faster capacities of spiral imaging. Imaging of the liver usually follows after a 30- to 45-s delay after injection. The technologist should be aware of the proper flow rates and protocols for intravenous contrasts before imaging.

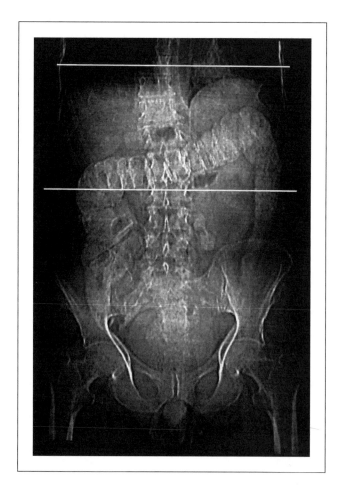

FIGURE 8-4

Coronal view (contrast study) of the liver with axial slices extending from the dome of the liver through the inferior border of the right lobe.

After the injection and appropriate delay of intravenous contrast medium, the second part of the scanning procedure begins. The second scanning procedure typically goes from the dome of the liver through the inferior border of the right lobe (Fig. 8-4).

CT IMAGING OF THE GASTROINTESTINAL TRACT

Elective minimum required is 3.

Common Indications

- Evaluation of abnormalities of alimentary canal

Imaging Considerations

PRE-EXAMINATION PREPARATION

Preparation for the abdominal CT examination may vary slightly for each imaging center or radiologist preference. The CT technologist must be aware of the specific protocol before scheduling the patient for an examination. Preparation of abdominal scanning typically begins the night before the actual imaging process. When the scan is to be completed the following morning, the patient will usually have a clear liquid supper the night before the examination and be NPO after midnight. If the CT scan is scheduled for the afternoon, the patient will consume a clear liquid supper and breakfast the day of the afternoon scan. The patient will be NPO after breakfast on the day of the afternoon scan. In either case of a morning or afternoon CT examination, the patient typically takes a laxative the evening before the scan. It is important that the patient understands that the presence of fecal matter can appear as a pathologic mass within the alimentary tract and restrict the flow of oral contrast medium.

ORAL CONTRAST ENHANCEMENT

Imaging of the abdomen normally is performed using a combination of oral and intravenous contrast media. Oral contrast media will differentiate the loops of bowel from a mass or an abnormal fluid collection. Two commonly used oral contrast agents are barium sulfate or water soluble based. The area of interest will determine the amount and time the contrast medium should be consumed. For example, when scanning the upper abdomen, the patient should consume approximately 400 mL of oral contrast medium 15 to 30 min in advance of the scanning. At the time of the scan, the patient will drink another 300 mL of contrast medium. For visualization of the lower abdomen and pelvis, the patient will consume 1200 mL of oral contrast medium 30 to 45 min before the scan, and another 300 mL of contrast is taken at the time of the scan. The purpose of the last 300 mL of contrast agent is to opacify the duodenum. The imaging facility and radiologist will dictate the type and timing for oral contrast medium.

INTRAVENOUS CONTRAST ENHANCEMENT

Intravenous contrast medium is used to enhance vascular and urinary structures of the abdomen and pelvis. It is the discretion of the imaging facility to determine the optimal injection rates and amounts of contrast to be used. It is the responsibility of the technologist to be familiar with all contraindications for the use of intravenous contrast medium. For vascular imaging of the gastrointestinal (GI) tract, facilities can use a single bolus injection followed by a delay before imaging. Another option is to use multiple bolus injections with different rates of flow. The technologist should be aware of the facility standards before using intravenous contrast.

There is controversy as to whether to perform an abdomen study with and without intravenous contrast medium or to perform a study with intravenous contrast alone. In cases for which there is a dual study, the noncontrast portion is completed first. The imaging of the noncontrast abdomen ranges from the xiphoid tip and extends to the iliac crest. If the pelvis is to be scanned as part of the abdomen study, the pelvis will be scanned during the second part of the study and will follow the injection of contrast medium. The second portion of the study will resume scanning at the xiphoid tip and continue through the symphysis pubis. When using intravenous contrast medium, it is important to determine the area of interest. This will designate the rate of contrast injection and the postinjection delay before the technologist starts to scan. The technologist should be aware of the facility standards when considering the imaging protocol.

Patient Preparations

The patient is placed supine and head first on the examination table with the midsagittal plane of the patient parallel with the longitudinal positioning lights. The midcoronal plane of the patient should pass through the center of the midhorizontal plane of the CT gantry. The patient's arms should be above the head. To minimize motion artifacts, the use of positioning pads and restraining straps should be considered. Foam padding placed under the patient's knees can relieve pressure on the lower back and add to the patient's comfort, which reduces the likelihood of patient motion. The patient should be informed of proper breathing techniques before the start of the examination. Thorough but simple instructions involving the imaging procedure will reduce patient motion. The decision to use conventional scanning or spiral scanning is determined by the imaging facility, with consideration to the patient's ability to remain motionless during the examination. The proper placement of radiation shielding is also an essential part of every CT examination.

Imaging Protocols

Imaging of the GI tract is not routinely completed as an individual examination. A routine CT examination of the abdomen and pelvis, with attention to the GI tract, is more of a typical examination process. The technologist may consider a thinner slice thickness to improve image quality when scanning the area of interest.

NONINTRAVENOUS CONTRAST STUDY OF THE GI TRACT

The first image produced is a coronal view of the abdomen. From the scout image, the technologist determines whether the midsagittal plane of the patient is centered relative to the long axis of the examination table. The range of axial images should extend from the dome of the liver through the rectum. The technologist selects a large FOV to accommodate the entire abdomen. The axial slices require no angulation of the gantry and should be perpendicular to the midsagittal plane of the patient (Fig. 8-5).

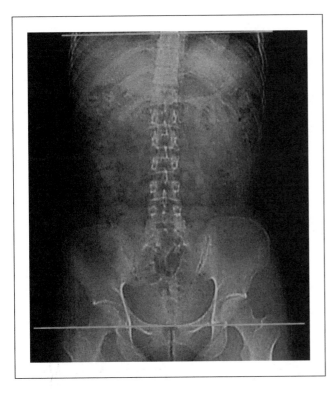

FIGURE 8-5

Coronal view of the gastrointestinal tract with axial slices extending from the dome of the liver through the rectum.

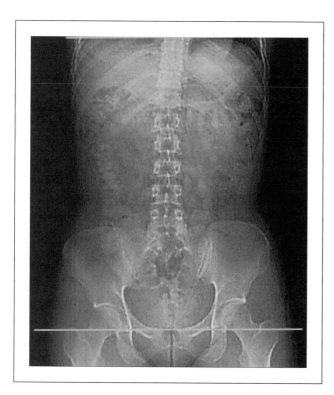

FIGURE 8-6

Coronal view (contrast study) of the gastro-intestinal tract with axial slices extending from the dome of the liver through the rectum.

INTRAVENOUS CONTRAST STUDY OF THE GI TRACT

Upon completion of the nonintravenous contrast study, the technologist repositions the patient at the beginning location of the diaphragm. When using conventional CT scanning of the GI tract, many facilities inject 100 to 150 mL of iodinated contrast at the rate of 1.5 to 2.0 mL/s. The remainder of intravenous contrast is injected at 1 mL/s. The second injection will continue to enhance the vasculature of the abdomen (Fig. 8-6).

If spiral scanning is the choice for abdominal imaging, the injection rate of 1.5 to 2.0 mL/s is used for the entire amount of contrast medium. This will accommodate for the faster capacities of spiral imaging. Imaging of the GI tract usually follows a 30- to 45-s delay after injection. The technologist should be aware of the proper flow rates and protocols for intravenous contrasts before imaging. After the injection and appropriate delay of intravenous contrast medium, the second part of the scanning procedure begins. The second scanning procedure typically goes from the dome of the liver through the rectum.

CT IMAGING OF THE PANCREAS

Mandatory minimum required is 5.

Common Indications

- Pancreatitis or jaundice
- Pancreatic cancer
- Evaluation of pancreatic pseudocyst

Imaging Considerations

PRE-EXAMINATION PREPARATION

Preparation for a pancreas CT examination may vary slightly for each imaging center or radiologist preference. The CT technologist must be aware of the specific protocol before scheduling the patient for an examination. Preparation for pancreas scanning begins the night before the actual imaging. If the CT scan is to be completed the following morning, the patient will have a clear liquid supper the night before the examination and be NPO after midnight. If the CT scan is scheduled for the afternoon, the patient will consume a clear liquid supper and breakfast the day of the afternoon scan. The patient will be NPO after breakfast on the day of the afternoon scan. In the case of morning or afternoon CT examination, the patient typically takes a laxative the evening before the scan. It is important that the patient understands that the presence of fecal matter can appear as a mass within the alimentary tract and restrict the flow of oral contrast medium.

ORAL CONTRAST ENHANCEMENT

Imaging of the pancreas normally is performed using a combination of oral and intravenous contrast media. Oral contrast medium will differentiate the loops of bowel from a mass or an abnormal fluid collection. In addition, oral contrast medium improves the definition of the border between the pancreatic head and the duodenum. Two commonly used oral contrast agents are barium sulfate or water soluble based. For opacification of the entire GI tract, the patient will consume 300 mL of oral contrast medium the night before the examination. Two hours before the examination, the patient should consume another 300 mL of oral contrast medium. As part of the imaging process, the patient will be required to drink 300 mL of oral contrast medium immediately before the examination. The purpose of the last 300 mL of contrast agent is to opacify the duodenum. The imaging facility dictates the type and timing for oral contrast medium.

INTRAVENOUS CONTRAST ENHANCEMENT

Intravenous contrast medium is used to enhance vascular and urinary structures of the abdomen and pelvis. It is the discretion of the imaging facility to determine the optimal injection rates and amounts of contrast to be used. It is the responsibility of the technologist to be familiar with all contraindications for the use of intravenous contrast medium. For vascular imaging of the pancreas, facilities can use a single bolus injection followed by a delay before imaging. Another option is to use multiple bolus injections with different rates of flow. The technologist should be aware of the facility standards before using intravenous contrast.

Patient Preparations

The patient is placed supine and head first on the examination table with the midsagittal plane of the patient parallel with the longitudinal positioning light. The midcoronal plane of the patient should pass through the center of the midhorizontal plane of the CT gantry. The patient's arms should be above the head. To minimize motion artifacts, the use of positioning pads and restraining straps should be considered. Foam padding placed under the patient's knees can relieve pressure on the lower back and add to the patient's comfort, which reduces the likelihood of patient motion. The patient should be informed of proper breathing techniques before the start of the examination. Thorough but simple instructions involving the imaging procedure will reduce patient motion. The decision to use conventional scanning or spiral scanning is determined by the imaging facility, with consideration to the patient's ability to remain motionless during the examination. The proper placement of radiation shielding is also an essential part of every CT examination.

Imaging Protocols

Imaging of the pancreas is not routinely completed as an individual examination. A routine CT examination of the abdomen and pelvis, with attention to the pancreas, is more of a typical examination process. The technologist may consider a thinner slice thickness to improve image quality when scanning the area of interest.

NONINTRAVENOUS CONTRAST STUDY OF THE PANCREAS

The first image produced is a coronal view of the abdomen. From the scout image, the technologist determines whether the midsagittal plane of the patient is centered relative to the long axis of the examination table. The range of axial images should extend from the dome of the liver through the iliac crest. The technologist selects a large FOV to accommodate the entire abdomen. The axial slices require no angulation of the gantry and should be perpendicular to the midsagittal plane of the patient (Fig. 8-7).

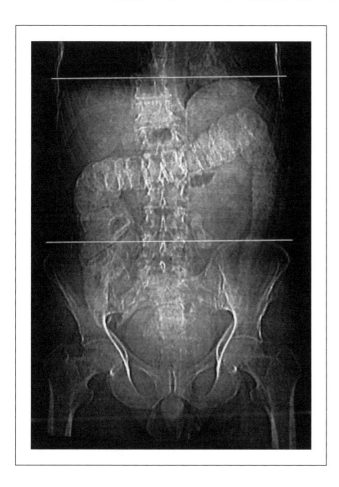

FIGURE 8-7

Coronal view of the pancreas with axial slices extending from the dome of the liver to the iliac crest.

INTRAVENOUS CONTRAST STUDY OF THE PANCREAS

Upon completion of the nonintravenous contrast study, the technologist repositions the patient at the beginning location of the diaphragm. When using conventional CT scanning of the pancreas, many facilities inject 100 to 150 mL of iodinated contrast at the rate of 1.5 to 2.0 mL/s. The remainder of intravenous contrast is injected at 1 mL/s. The second injection will continue to enhance the vasculature of the abdomen (Fig. 8-8).

If spiral scanning is the choice for abdominal imaging, the injection rate of 1.5 to 2.0 mL/s is used for the entire amount of contrast medium. This will accommodate for the faster capabilities of spiral imaging. Imaging of the pancreas usually follows a 20- to 30-s delay after injection. The technologist should be aware of the proper flow rates and protocols for intravenous contrasts before imaging. After the injection and appropriate delay of intravenous contrast medium, the second part of the scanning procedure begins. The second scanning procedure typically goes from the dome of the liver to the iliac crest.

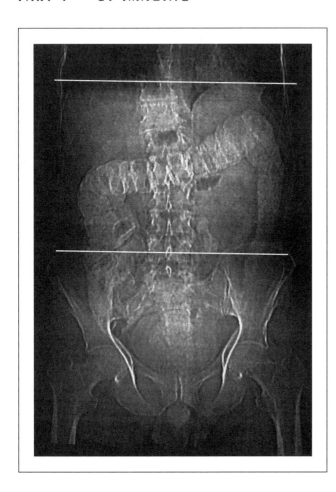

FIGURE 8-8
Coronal view of the pancreas with axial slices extending from the dome of the liver to the iliac crest.

CT IMAGING OF THE ADRENALS

Elective minimum required is 3.

Common Indications

- Adrenal cortex carcinoma
- Pheochromocytomas
- Adrenal gland hyperplasia

Imaging Considerations

PRE-EXAMINATION PREPARATION

Preparation for an adrenal CT examination may vary slightly for each imaging center or radiologist preference. The CT technologist must be aware of the specific protocol before scheduling the patient for an examination. Preparation for adrenal scanning begins the night before the actual imaging. If the CT scan is to be completed the following morning, the patient will have a clear liquid supper the night before the examination and be NPO after midnight. If the CT scan is scheduled for the afternoon, the patient will consume a clear liquid supper and breakfast the day of the afternoon scan. The patient will be NPO after breakfast on the day of the afternoon scan. In the case of morning or afternoon CT examination, the patient typically takes a laxative the evening before the scan. It is important that the patient understands that the presence of fecal matter can appear as a mass within the alimentary tract and restrict the flow of oral contrast medium.

ORAL CONTRAST ENHANCEMENT

Imaging of the adrenals normally is perfomed using a combination of oral and intravenous contrast media. Oral contrast medium will differentiate the loops of bowel from a mass or an abnormal fluid collection. Two commonly used oral contrast agents are barium sulfate or water soluble based. For opacification of the entire GI tract, the patient will consume 300 mL of oral contrast medium the night before the examination. Two hours before the examination, the patient should consume another 300 mL of oral contrast medium. As part of the imaging process, the patient is required to drink 300 mL of oral contrast medium immediately before the examination. The purpose of the last 300 mL of contrast agent is to opacify the duodenum. The imaging facility dictates the type and timing for oral contrast medium.

INTRAVENOUS CONTRAST ENHANCEMENT

Intravenous contrast medium is used to enhance vascular and urinary structures of the abdomen and pelvis. It is the discretion of the imaging facility to determine the optimal injection rates and amounts of contrast to be used. It is the responsibility of the technologist to be familiar with all contraindications for the use of intravenous contrast medium. For vascular imaging of the adrenals, facilities can use a single bolus injection followed by a delay before imaging. Another option is to use multiple bolus injections with different rates of flow. The technologist should be aware of the facility standards before using intravenous contrast.

Patient Preparations

The patient is placed supine and head first on the examination table with the midsagittal plane of the patient parallel with the longitudinal positioning light. The midcoronal plane of the patient should pass through the center of the midhorizontal plane of the CT gantry. The patient's arms should be above the head. To minimize motion artifacts, the use of positioning pads and restraining straps should be considered. Foam padding placed under the patient's knees can relieve pressure on the lower back and add to the patient's comfort, which reduces the likelihood of patient motion. The patient should be informed of proper breathing techniques before the start of the examination.

Thorough but simple instructions involving the imaging procedure will reduce patient motion. The decision to use conventional scanning or spiral scanning is determined by the imaging facility, with consideration to the patient's ability to remain motionless during the examination. The proper placement of radiation shielding is also an essential part of every CT examination.

Imaging Protocols

Imaging of the adrenal is not routinely completed as an individual examination. A routine CT examination of the abdomen and pelvis, with attention to the adrenals, is more of a typical examination process. The technologist may consider a thinner slice thickness to improve image quality when scanning the area of interest.

NONINTRAVENOUS CONTRAST STUDY OF THE ADRENALS

The first image produced is a coronal view of the abdomen. From the scout image, the technologist determines whether the midsagittal plane of the patient is centered relative to the long axis of the examination table. The range of axial images should extend from the dome of the liver to the iliac crest. The technologist selects a large FOV to

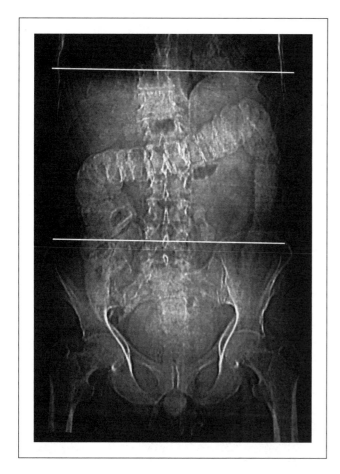

FIGURE 8-9

Coronal view of the adrenals with axial slices extending from the dome of the liver to the iliac crest.

accommodate the entire abdomen. The axial slices require no angulation of the gantry and should be perpendicular to the midsagittal plane of the patient (Fig. 8-9).

INTRAVENOUS CONTRAST STUDY OF THE ADRENALS

Upon completion of the nonintravenous contrast study, the technologist repositions the patient at the beginning location of the diaphragm. When using conventional CT scanning of the adrenals, many facilities inject 100 to 150 mL of iodinated contrast at the rate of 1.5 to 2.0 mL/s. The remainder of intravenous contrast is injected at 1 mL/s. The second injection will continue to enhance the vasculature of the abdomen.

If spiral scanning is the choice for abdominal imaging, the injection rate of 1.5 to 2.0 mL/s is used for the entire amount of contrast medium. This will accommodate for the faster capacities of spiral imaging. Imaging of the adrenals usually follows a 60-s delay after injection. The technologist should be aware of the proper flow rates and protocols for intravenous contrasts before imaging. After the injection and appropriate delay of intravenous contrast medium, the second part of the scanning procedure begins. The second scanning procedure typically goes from the dome of the liver to the iliac crest (Fig. 8-10).

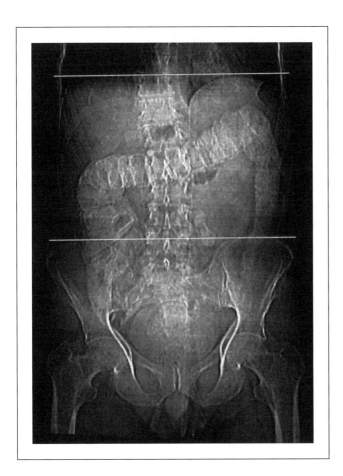

FIGURE 8-10

Coronal view of the adrenals with axial slices extending from the dome of the liver to the iliac crest.

CT IMAGING OF THE KIDNEYS

Mandatory minimum required is 5.

Common Indications

- Evaluation of renal cysts
- Evaluation of renal masses and metastases
- Evaluation of abscesses and arterial venous malformations

Imaging Considerations

PRE-EXAMINATION PREPARATION

Preparation for a kidney CT examination may vary slightly for each imaging center or radiologist preference. The CT technologist must be aware of the specific protocol before scheduling the patient for an examination. Preparation for kidney scanning begins the night before the actual imaging. If the CT scan is to be completed the following morning, the patient will have a clear liquid supper the night before the examination and be NPO after midnight. If the CT scan is scheduled for the afternoon, the patient will consume a clear liquid supper and breakfast the day of the afternoon scan. The patient will be NPO after breakfast on the day of the afternoon scan. In the case of morning or afternoon CT examination, the patient typically takes a laxative the evening before the scan. It is important that the patient understands that the presence of fecal matter can appear as a mass within the alimentary tract and restrict the flow of oral contrast medium.

ORAL CONTRAST ENHANCEMENT

Imaging of the kidneys normally is performed using a combination of oral and intravenous contrast media. Oral contrast medium will differentiate the loops of bowel from a mass or an abnormal fluid collection. Two commonly used oral contrast agents are barium sulfate or water soluble based. For opacification of the entire GI tract, the patient will consume 300 mL of oral contrast medium the night before the examination. Two hours before the examination, the patient should consume another 300 mL of oral contrast medium. As part of the imaging process, the patient is required to drink 300 mL of oral contrast medium immediately before the examination. The purpose of the last 300 mL of contrast agent is to opacify the duodenum. The imaging facility dictates the type and timing for oral contrast medium.

INTRAVENOUS CONTRAST ENHANCEMENT

Intravenous contrast medium is used to enhance vascular and urinary structures of the abdomen and pelvis. It is the discretion of the imaging facility to determine the optimal injection rates and amounts of contrast to be used. It is the responsibility of the technologist to be familiar with all contraindications for the use of intravenous contrast medium. For vascular imaging of the kidneys, facilities can use a single bolus injection followed by a delay before imaging. Another option is to use multiple bolus injections with different rates of flow. The technologist should be aware of the facility standards before using intravenous contrast.

Patient Preparations

The patient is placed supine and head first on the examination table with the midsagittal plane of the patient parallel with the longitudinal positioning lights. The midcoronal plane of the patient should pass through the center of the midhorizontal plane of the CT gantry. The patient's arms should be above the head. To minimize motion artifacts, the use of positioning pads and restraining straps should be considered. Foam padding placed under the patient's knees can relieve pressure on the lower back and add to the patient's comfort, which reduces the likelihood of patient motion. The patient should be informed of proper breathing techniques before the start of the examination. Thorough but simple instructions involving the imaging procedure will reduce patient motion. The decision to use conventional scanning or spiral scanning is determined by the imaging facility, with consideration to the patient's ability to remain motionless during the examination. The proper placement of radiation shielding is also an essential part of every CT examination.

Imaging Protocols

Imaging of the kidneys is not routinely completed as an individual examination. A routine CT examination of the abdomen and pelvis, with attention to the kidneys, is more of a typical examination process. The technologist may consider a thinner slice thickness through the area of interest to improve image quality.

NONINTRAVENOUS CONTRAST STUDY OF THE KIDNEYS

The first image produced is a coronal view of the abdomen. From the scout image, the technologist determines whether the midsagittal plane of the patient is centered relative to the long axis of the examination table. The range of axial images should extend from the dome of the liver to the iliac crest. The technologist selects a large FOV to accommodate the entire abdomen. The axial slices require no angulation of the gantry and should be perpendicular to the midsagittal plane of the patient (Fig. 8-11).

INTRAVENOUS CONTRAST STUDY OF THE KIDNEYS

Upon completion of the nonintravenous contrast study, the technologist repositions the patient at the beginning location of the diaphragm. When using conventional CT scanning of the kidneys,

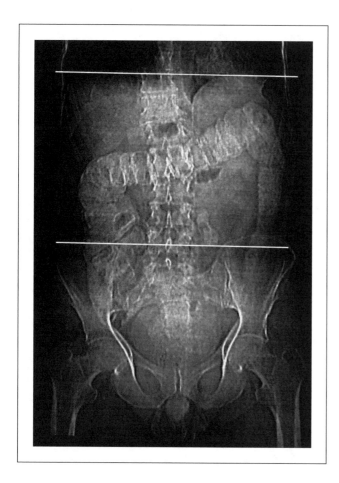

FIGURE 8-11

Coronal view of the kidneys with axial slices extending from the dome of the liver to the iliac crest.

many facilities inject 100 to 150 mL of iodinated contrast at the rate of 1.5 to 2.0 mL/s. The remainder of intravenous contrast is injected at 1 mL/s. This second of dual injections will continue to enhance the vasculature of the abdomen.

If spiral scanning is the choice for abdominal imaging, the injection rate of 1.5 to 2.0 mL/s is used for the entire amount of contrast medium. This will accommodate for the faster capacities of spiral imaging. Imaging of the kidneys usually follows a 60-s delay after injection. The technologist should be aware of the proper flow rates and protocols for intravenous contrasts before imaging. After the injection and appropriate delay of intravenous contrast medium, the second part of the scanning procedure begins. The second scanning procedure typically goes from the dome of the liver to the iliac crest (Fig. 8-12).

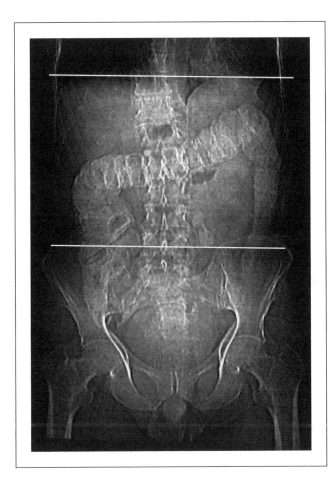

FIGURE 8-12

Coronal view of the kidneys with axial slices extending from the dome of the liver to the iliac crest.

CT VASCULAR IMAGING OF THE ABDOMEN

Mandatory minimum required is 5.

Common Indications

- Evaluation of aneurysms and dissections of the abdominal vasculature
- Evaluation of branches of the abdominal aorta
- Evaluation of portal circulation
- Evaluation of inferior vena cava

Imaging Considerations

PRE-EXAMINATION PREPARATION

Preparation for an abdominal vascular CT examination may vary slightly for each imaging center or radiologist preference. The CT technologist must be aware of the specific protocol before scheduling the patient for an examination. Preparation of abdominal scanning begins the night before the actual imaging. If the examination is to be completed the following morning, the patient will have a clear liquid supper the night before and be NPO after midnight. If the CT examination is scheduled for the afternoon, the patient will consume a clear liquid supper and breakfast. The patient will be NPO after breakfast on the day of the afternoon scan. In either case, the patient typically takes a laxative the evening before the scan. It is important that the patient understand that the presence of fecal matter can appear as a mass within the alimentary tract and restrict the flow of oral contrast medium.

ORAL CONTRAST ENHANCEMENT

Imaging of the vascular structures of the abdomen normally is performed using a combination of oral and intravenous contrast media. Oral contrast medium will differentiate the loops of bowel from a mass or an abnormal fluid collection. Two commonly used oral contrast agents are barium sulfate or water soluble based. The area of interest will determine the amount and time of consumption of oral contrast medium. For example, when scanning the upper abdomen, the patient should consume approximately 400 mL of oral contrast medium 15 to 30 min in advance of the scanning. At the time of the scan, the patient will drink another 300 mL of contrast medium. For visualization of the lower abdomen and pelvis, the patient will consume 1200 mL of oral contrast medium 30 to 45 min before the scan and another 300 mL of contrast at the time of the scan. The purpose of the last 300 mL of contrast agent is to opacify the duodenum. The imaging facility dictates the type and timing for oral contrast medium.

INTRAVENOUS CONTRAST ENHANCEMENT

Imaging the vascular structures of the abdomen normally requires the use of intravenous contrast medium. Intravenous contrast medium is used to enhance vascular structures such as the portal vein, abdominal aorta and inferior vena cava, and iliac arteries and veins. In addition, the use of intravenous contrast medium is used for the visualization of the ureters and bladder. It is the discretion of the imaging facility to determine the optimal injection rates and amounts of contrast to be used. It is the responsibility of the technologist to be familiar with all contraindications for the use of intravenous contrast medium. For vascular imaging of the abdomen, some facilities use a single bolus injection followed by a delay before imaging. Other facilities may use multiple bolus injections with different rates of flow. The technologist should be aware of the facility standards before using intravenous contrast.

There is controversy as to whether to perform an abdomen study with and without intravenous contrast medium or to perform a study with intravenous contrast alone. In cases for which there is a dual study, the noncontrast portion is completed first. The imaging of the noncontrast abdomen ranges from the xiphoid tip and extends to the iliac crest. If the pelvis is to be scanned as part of the abdomen study, it will be scanned during the second part of the study, which will include the contrast injection. The second portion of the study will resume scanning at the xiphoid tip and continue through the symphysis pubis. When using intravenous contrast, it is important to determine the area of interest. This will designate the rate of contrast injection and the postinjection delay before imaging begins. The technologist should be aware of the facility standards when considering the imaging protocol.

Patient Preparations

The patient is placed supine and head first on the examination table with the midsagittal plane of the patient parallel with the longitudinal positioning lights. The midcoronal plane of the patient should pass through the center of the midhorizontal plane of the CT gantry. The patient's arms should be above the head. To minimize motion artifacts, the use of positioning pads and restraining straps should be considered. Foam padding placed under the patient's knees can relieve pressure on the lower back and add to the patient's comfort, which reduces the likelihood of patient motion. The patient should be informed of proper breathing techniques before the start of the examination. Thorough but simple instructions involving the imaging procedure will also reduce patient motion. The decision to use conventional scanning or spiral scanning is determined by the imaging facility, with consideration to the patient's ability to remain motionless during the examination. The proper placement of radiation shielding is also an essential part of every CT examination.

Imaging Protocols

NONINTRAVENOUS CONTRAST STUDY OF THE ABDOMEN

The first image produced is a coronal view of the abdomen. From the scout image, the technologist determines whether the midsagittal plane of the patient is centered relative to the long axis of the examination table. The range of axial images should extend from the xiphoid tip through the level of the iliac crest. The technologist selects a large FOV to accommodate the entire abdomen. The axial slices do not require angulation of the gantry and should be perpendicular to the midsagittal plane of the patient (Fig. 8-13).

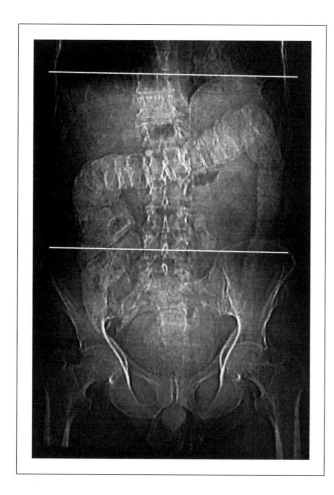

FIGURE 8-13

Coronal view of the abdomen with axial slices extending from the xiphoid tip through the level of the iliac crest.

INTRAVENOUS CONTRAST STUDY OF THE ABDOMEN

Upon completion of the nonintravenous contrast study, the technologist repositions the patient at the beginning location of the xiphoid tip. With conventional CT scanning of the abdomen, many facilities inject 100 to 150 mL of iodinated contrast injected at 1.5 to 2.0 mL/s. The remainder of intravenous contrast is injected at 1 mL/s. This method of dual injection rates will continue to enhance the vasculature of the abdomen. When spiral scanning is the choice for abdominal imaging, the rate of injection is 1.5 to 2.0 mL/s for the entire amount of contrast medium. The single bolus injection will accommodate for the faster capacities of spiral imaging. The technologist should be aware of the proper flow rates and protocols for intravenous injections of the facility before imaging. After the injection and appropriate delay of intravenous contrast medium, the second part of the scanning procedure begins. The second scanning procedure typically goes from the xiphoid tip through the symphysis. The choice of CT scanner may require a delay following the range from the xiphoid tip to the adrenal glands. This delay will allow for the contrast medium to reach the patient's kidneys. After a second delay, the technologist can complete the study by scanning the range from the

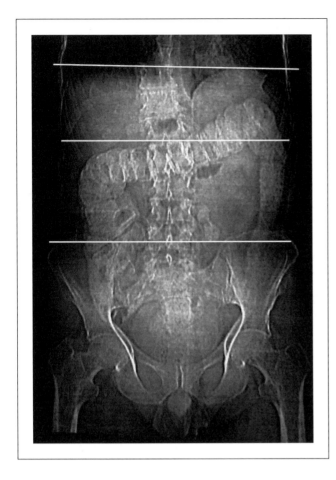

FIGURE 8-14

Coronal view (contrast study) of the abdomen with axial slices extending from the xiphoid tip to the adrenals. The second range is from the adrenals through the symphysis pubis.

adrenal glands through the bladder. The selection of delay times and separate scan ranges is dependent on the imaging facility (Fig. 8-14).

CT IMAGING OF THE PELVIS

Mandatory minimum required is 5.

Common Indications

- Staging of masses, tumors, and lesions within the pelvis
- Evaluation of bladder and rectum
- Evaluation of the response of tissue after therapy

Imaging Considerations

PRE-EXAMINATION PREPARATION

Preparation for a CT examination of the pelvis may vary slightly for each imaging center or radiologist preference. The CT technologist must be aware of the specific protocol before scheduling the patient for an examination. Preparation for pelvis scanning begins the night before the actual imaging. If the CT scan is to be completed the following morning, the patient will have a clear liquid supper the night before the examination and be NPO after midnight. If the CT scan is scheduled for the afternoon, the patient will consume a clear liquid supper and breakfast the day of the afternoon scan. The patient will be NPO after breakfast on the day of the afternoon scan. In the case of morning or afternoon CT examination, the patient typically takes a laxative the evening before the scan. It is important that the patient understands that the presence of fecal matter can appear as a mass within the alimentary tract and restrict the flow of oral contrast medium.

ORAL CONTRAST ENHANCEMENT

Imaging of the pelvis normally is performed using a combination of oral, rectal, and intravenous contrast media. Oral contrast medium will differentiate the loops of bowel from a mass or an abnormal fluid collection. Two commonly used oral contrast agents are barium sulfate or water soluble based. For opacification of the entire GI tract, the patient will consume 300 mL of oral contrast medium the night before the examination. Two hours before the examination, the patient should consume another 300 mL of oral contrast medium. As part of the imaging process, the patient is required to drink 300 mL of oral contrast medium immediately before the examination. The purpose of the last 300 mL of contrast agent is to opacify the duodenum. Contrast medium may be introduced by enema to visualize the rectum and distal portion of the descending colon. The imaging facility dictates the type and timing for oral contrast medium, as well as the amount and use of contrast medium administrated as an enema.

INTRAVENOUS CONTRAST ENHANCEMENT

Intravenous contrast medium is used to enhance vascular and urinary structures of the abdomen and pelvis. It is the discretion of the imaging facility to determine the optimal injection rates and amounts of contrast to be used. For vascular imaging of the pelvis, facilities can use a single bolus injection followed by a delay before imaging. Another option is to use multiple bolus injections with different rates of flow. The technologist should be aware of the facility standards before using intravenous contrast.

Patient Preparations

The patient is placed supine and head first on the examination table with the midsagittal plane of the patient parallel with the longitudinal positioning light. The midcoronal plane of the patient should pass through the center of the midhorizontal plane of the CT gantry. The patient's arms should be above the head. To minimize motion artifacts, the use of positioning pads and restraining straps should be considered. Foam padding placed under the patient's knees can relieve pressure on the lower back and add to the patient's comfort, which reduces the likelihood of patient motion. The patient should be informed of proper breathing techniques before the start of the examination. Thorough but simple instructions involving the imaging procedure will reduce patient motion. The decision to use conventional scanning or spiral scanning is determined by the imaging facility, with consideration to the patient's ability to remain motionless during the examination. The proper placement of radiation shielding is also an essential part of every CT examination.

Imaging Protocols

Imaging of the pelvis is not routinely completed as an individual examination. A routine CT examination of the abdomen and pelvis, with attention to the pelvis, is more of a typical examination process. The technologist may consider a thinner slice thickness to improve image quality when scanning the area of interest.

NONINTRAVENOUS CONTRAST STUDY OF THE PELVIS

The first image produced is a coronal view of the abdomen. From the scout image, the technologist determines whether the midsagittal plane of the patient is centered relative to the long axis of the examination table. The range of axial images should extend from the iliac crest through the symphysis pubis. The technologist selects a large

FIGURE 8-15

Coronal view of the pelvis with axial slices extending from the iliac crest through the symphysis pubis.

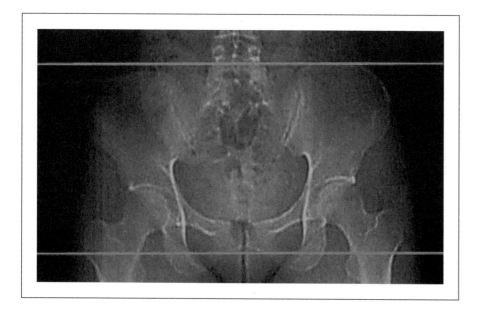

FOV to accommodate the entire pelvis. The axial slices require no angulation of the gantry and should be perpendicular to the midsagittal plane of the patient (Fig. 8-15).

INTRAVENOUS CONTRAST STUDY OF THE PELVIS

Upon completion of the nonintravenous contrast study, the technologist repositions the patient at the beginning location of the iliac crest. When using conventional CT scanning of the pelvis, many facilities inject 100 to 150 mL of iodinated contrast at the rate of 1.5 to 2.0 mL/s. The remainder of intravenous contrast is injected at 1 mL/s. This second of dual injections will continue to enhance the vasculature of the abdominal and pelvic structures.

If spiral scanning is the choice for pelvic imaging, the injection rate of 1.5 to 2.0 mL/s is used for the entire amount of contrast medium. This will accommodate for the faster capacities of spiral imaging. Imaging of the pelvis usually follows a delay after injection. This delay is dependent on the anatomy of interest. For example, for visualization of the bladder, the delay can be a few minutes after the intravenous injection. The technologist should be aware of the proper flow rates and protocols for intravenous contrasts before imaging. After the injection and appropriate delay of intravenous contrast medium, the second part of the scanning procedure begins. The second scanning procedure typically goes from the iliac crest through the symphysis pubis (Fig. 8-16).

FIGURE 8-16

Coronal view of the pelvis with axial slices extending from the iliac crest through the symphysis pubis.

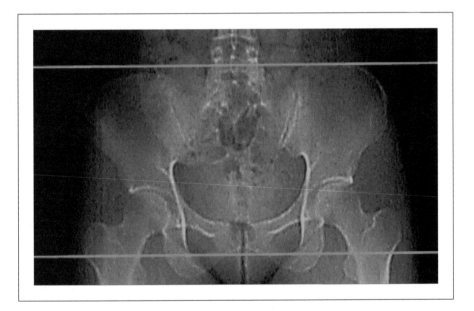

CHAPTER 9

CT Imaging Procedures of the Musculoskeletal System

The protocol marked with an asterisk must be completed on a patient, not a simulation.

	Mandatory	Elective
Musculoskeletal System		
Upper extremity	5	
Lower extremity	5	
Pelvic girdle and hips*	5*	
After arthrography		3

CT MUSCULOSKELETAL EXAMINATION OF THE SHOULDER

Mandatory minimum required is 5.

Common Indications

- Evaluation of joints, bones, and soft tissues in the musculoskeletal system
- Demonstration of bone and soft tissue lesions

Imaging Considerations

Each examination for upper extremities of the musculoskeletal system is customized to the individual's specific clinical history. The technologist should consider symmetry at all times when positioning the patient for the specific examination. When possible, simultaneous visualization of both extremities is diagnostically important for comparison. The upper extremities are typically scanned with the patient supine and head first into the scanner. Some facilities require both lateral and coronal scouts to determine the range of cross-sectional slices. The slices within the scan range should be set accordingly. With CT examination of upper extremities, the slice thickness is a collaborative effort between the patient's abilities and the radiologist's diagnostic needs. Thin slices will improve spatial resolution; therefore, thin slices are used for evaluation of small masses or fractures, whereas large masses can be demonstrated with thicker slices.

Imaging of musculoskeletal upper extremities is usually completed with the image plane being perpendicular to the region of interest. The scan FOV should be large enough to include both extremities simultaneously, to serve as a comparison of normal anatomy. After the scan, the technologist can reconstruct the individual image in the appropriate FOV. Three-dimensional reconstructions may be helpful for surgical planning of the extremity.

Intravenous contrast medium is not typically used, but in specific cases may be useful for evaluation of the vascularity of the tumor. Contrast medium should be used according to facility standards. In cases of a postarthrogram CT examination, the use of iodinated contrast medium, air, or both, may be injected into the joint capsule.

The decision to use conventional or spiral scanning is determined by the imaging facility, with consideration to the patient's ability to remain motionless during the examination. An accurate explanation of the examination process before the examination and consideration to patient comfort will reduce voluntary motion during the imaging process.

Patient Preparations

The patient is placed supine and head first on the examination table. The patient is positioned with the midsagittal plane of the patient parallel with the longitudinal positioning light. The technologist should use positioning pads and restraining straps as needed. The technologist should have the patient relax the shoulders in a comfortable position. The patient should place the arms beside the abdomen. To minimize motion artifacts, the use of restraining straps and positioning cushions should be considered. Foam padding placed under the patient's knees can relieve pressure on the lower back and add to the patient's comfort, which reduces the likelihood of patient motion. Thorough but simple instructions involving the imaging procedure will also reduce patient motion. The proper placement of radiation shielding is also an essential part of every CT examination.

Imaging Protocols

AXIAL IMAGES OF THE SHOULDER

The first image produced is a coronal view of the upper chest. From the scout image, the technologist determines whether the midsagittal plane of the patient is centered relative to the long axis of the examination table. The axial slices should be perpendicular to the midsagittal plane of the body and without angulation of the gantry. The range of slices should extend from the acromion through the sternoclavicular joints (Fig. 9-1).

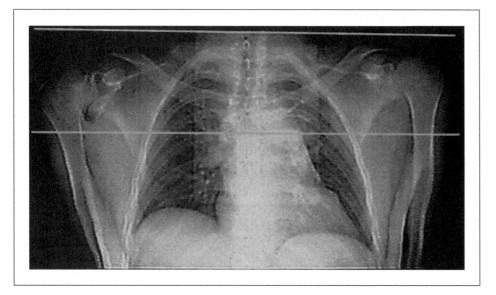

FIGURE 9-1

Anteroposterior view of shoulder to show proper centering and alignment. Lines should extend from the acromion through the sternoclavicular joints.

CT MUSCULOSKELETAL EXAMINATION OF THE ELBOW

Mandatory minimum required is 5.

Common Indications

- Evaluation of joints, bones, and soft tissues in the musculoskeletal system
- Demonstration of bone and soft tissue lesions

Imaging Considerations

Each examination for upper extremities of the musculoskeletal system is customized to the individual's specific clinical history. The technologist should consider symmetry at all times when positioning the patient for the specific examination. When possible, simultaneous visualization of both extremities is diagnostically important for comparison. The upper extremities can be scanned with the patient supine or prone and head first into the scanner. Some facilities require both lateral and coronal scouts to determine the range of cross-sectional slices. The slices within the scan range should be set accordingly. Thin slices will improve spatial resolution; therefore, thin slices are used for evaluation of small masses or fractures, whereas large masses can be demonstrated with thicker slices.

Imaging of musculoskeletal upper extremities is usually completed with the image plane being perpendicular to the region of interest. Three-dimensional reconstructions may be helpful for surgical planning of the extremity.

Intravenous contrast medium is not typically used, but in specific cases may be useful for evaluation of the vascularity of the tumor. Contrast medium should be used according to facility standards. In cases of a postarthrogram CT examination, the use of iodinated contrast medium, air, or both, may be injected into the joint capsule.

The decision to use conventional or spiral scanning is determined by the imaging facility, with consideration to the patient's ability to remain motionless during the examination. An accurate explanation of the examination process and consideration to patient comfort will reduce voluntary motion during the imaging process.

Patient Preparations

The patient is placed supine or prone and head first on the examination table. The patient is positioned with the midsagittal plane of the arm parallel with the longitudinal positioning lights. The patient's arm is extended above the head. The technologist should use positioning pads and restraining straps as needed. If the patient is in the supine position, foam padding placed under the arm will support the arm in a parallel position to the table and prevent distortion of axial images. If the patient is supine, foam padding placed under the patient's knees can relieve pressure on the lower back and add to the patient's comfort, which reduces the likelihood of patient motion. For prone positioning, the technologist should place foam padding under the patient's ankles to assist in patient comfort. Thorough but simple instructions involving the imaging procedure will also reduce patient motion. Proper placement of radiation shielding is also an essential part of every CT examination.

Imaging Protocols

AXIAL IMAGES OF THE ELBOW

The first image produced will be a coronal or lateral view of the elbow. From the scout image, the technologist determines whether the midsagittal plane of the patient's humerus is parallel with the long axis of the examination table. The axial slices should be perpendicular to the midsagittal plane of the elbow (Fig. 9-2).

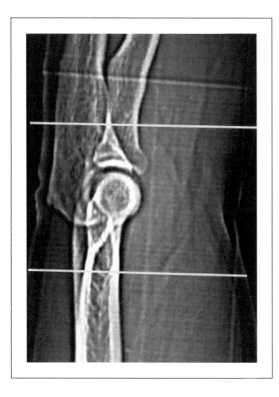

FIGURE 9-2

Demonstration of the elbow to show proper centering and alignment. Lines should extend from an area superior to and through the elbow joint.

CT MUSCULOSKELETAL EXAMINATION OF THE WRIST

Mandatory minimum required is 5.

Common Indications

- Evaluation of joints, bones, and soft tissues in the musculoskeletal system
- Demonstration of bone and soft tissue lesions

Imaging Considerations

Each examination for upper extremities of the musculoskeletal system is customized to the individual's specific clinical history. The technologist should consider symmetry at all times when positioning the patient for the specific examination. When possible, simultaneous visualization of both extremities is diagnostically important for comparison. The upper extremities can be scanned with the patient supine or prone and head first into the scanner. Some facilities require both lateral and coronal scouts to determine the range of cross-sectional slices. The slices within the scan range should be set

101

accordingly. With CT examination of upper extremities, the slice thickness is a collaborative effort between the patient's abilities and the radiologist's diagnostic needs. Thin slices will improve spatial resolution; therefore, thin slices are used for evaluation of small masses or fractures, whereas large masses can be demonstrated with thicker slices.

Imaging of musculoskeletal upper extremities is usually completed with the image plane being perpendicular to the region of interest. The scan FOV should be large enough to include both extremities simultaneously, to serve as a comparison of normal anatomy. After the scan, the technologist can reconstruct the individual image in the appropriate FOV. Three-dimensional reconstructions may be helpful for surgical planning of the extremity.

Intravenous contrast medium is not typically used, but in specific cases may be useful for evaluation of the vascularity of the tumor. Contrast medium should be used according to facility standards. In cases of a postarthrogram CT examination, the use of iodinated contrast medium, air, or both may be injected into the joint capsule.

The decision to use conventional or spiral scanning is determined by the imaging facility, with consideration to the patient's ability to remain motionless during the examination. An accurate explanation of the examination process before the examination and consideration to patient comfort will reduce voluntary motion during the imaging process.

Patient Preparations

The patient is placed supine or prone and head first on the examination table. The patient is positioned with the midsagittal plane of the patient parallel with the longitudinal positioning light. The patient's arms are extended above the head. The technologist should use positioning pads and restraining straps as needed. If the patient is supine, foam padding placed under the patient's knees can relieve pressure on the lower back and add to the patient's comfort, which reduces the likelihood of patient motion. For prone positioning, the technologist should place foam padding under the patient's ankles to assist in patient comfort. Thorough but simple instructions involving the imaging procedure will also reduce patient motion. The proper placement of radiation shielding is also an essential part of every CT examination.

Imaging Protocols

AXIAL IMAGES OF THE WRIST

The first image produced can be a coronal or lateral view of the wrist. From the scout image, the technologist determines whether the patient's wrist is parallel with the long axis of the examination table. The axial slices should be perpendicular to the sagittal plane of the wrist (Fig. 9-3).

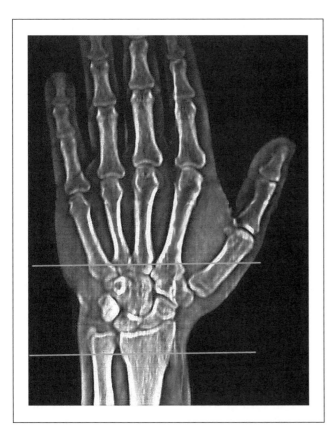

FIGURE 9-3

Anteroposterior view of the wrist to show proper centering and alignment. Lines should extend from and through the carpals.

CT MUSCULOSKELETAL EXAMINATION OF THE KNEE

Mandatory minimum required is 5.

Common Indications

- Evaluation of joints, bones, and soft tissues in the musculoskeletal system
- Demonstration of bone and soft tissue lesions

Imaging Considerations

Each examination for lower extremities of the musculoskeletal system is customized to the individual's specific clinical history. The technologist should consider symmetry at all times when positioning the patient for the specific examination. When possible, simultaneous

103

visualization of both extremities is diagnostically important for comparison. The lower extremities are typically scanned with the patient supine and feet first into the scanner. Some facilities require both lateral and coronal scouts to determine the range of cross-sectional slices. The slices within the scan range should be set accordingly. With CT examination of upper extremities, the slice thickness is a collaborative effort between the patient's abilities and the radiologist's diagnostic needs. Thin slices will improve spatial resolution; therefore, thin slices are used for evaluation of small masses or fractures, whereas large masses can be demonstrated with thicker slices.

Imaging of musculoskeletal lower extremities is usually completed with the image plane being perpendicular to the region of interest. The scan FOV should be large enough to include both extremities simultaneously, to serve as a comparison of normal anatomy. After the scan, the technologist can reconstruct the individual image in the appropriate FOV. Three-dimensional reconstructions may be helpful for surgical planning of the extremity.

Intravenous contrast medium is not typically used, but in specific cases may be useful for evaluation of the vascularity of the tumor. Contrast medium should be used according to facility standards. In cases of a postarthrogram CT examination, the use of iodinated contrast medium, air, or both, may be injected into the joint capsule.

The decision to use conventional or spiral scanning is determined by the imaging facility, with consideration to the patient's ability to remain motionless during the examination. An accurate explanation of the examination process before the examination and consideration to patient comfort will reduce voluntary motion during the imaging process.

Patient Preparations

The patient is placed supine and feet first on the examination table. The patient is positioned with the midsagittal plane of the patient parallel with the longitudinal positioning light. The patient's arms should be across the abdomen or along the sides of the patient. The technologist should use positioning pads and restraining straps as needed. If the patient is supine, foam padding placed under the patient's knees can relieve pressure on the lower back and add to the patient's comfort, which reduces the likelihood of patient motion. Thorough but simple instructions involving the imaging procedure will also reduce patient motion. The proper placement of radiation shielding is also an essential part of every CT examination.

Imaging Protocols

AXIAL IMAGES OF THE KNEES

The first image produced will be a coronal view of the knee. From the scout image, the technologist determines whether the sagittal plane of the patient's knees are parallel with the long axis of the examination

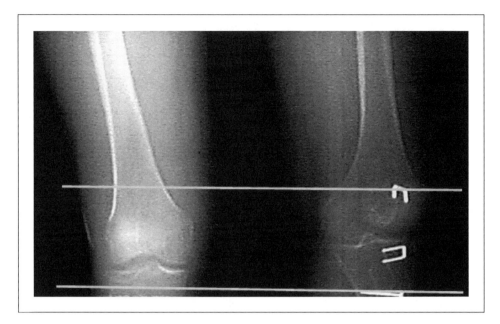

FIGURE 9-4

Anteroposterior view of the knee to show proper centering and alignment. Lines should extend from an area superior to and through the knee joint.

table. The axial slices should be perpendicular to the midsagittal plane of the knee (Fig. 9-4).

CT MUSCULOSKELETAL EXAMINATION OF THE ANKLE AND FOOT

Mandatory minimum required is 5.

Common Indications

- Evaluation of joints, bones, and soft tissues in the musculoskeletal system
- Demonstration of bone and soft tissue lesions

Imaging Considerations

Each examination for lower extremities of the musculoskeletal system is customized to the individual's specific clinical history. The technologist should consider symmetry at all times when positioning the patient for the specific examination. When possible, simultaneous visualization of both extremities is diagnostically important for comparison. The lower extremities are typically scanned with the patient supine and feet first into the scanner. Some facilities require both lateral and coronal scouts to determine the range of cross-sectional slices. The slices within the scan range should be set accordingly. With CT examination of upper extremities, the slice thickness is a collaborative effort between the patient's abilities and the radiologist's diagnostic needs. Thin slices will improve spatial resolution; therefore, thin slices are used for evaluation of small masses or fractures, whereas large masses can be demonstrated with thicker slices.

Imaging of musculoskeletal lower extremities is usually completed with the image plane being perpendicular to the region of interest. The scan FOV should be large enough to include both extremities simultaneously, to serve as a comparison of normal anatomy. After the scan, the technologist can reconstruct the individual image in the appropriate FOV. Three-dimensional reconstructions may be helpful for surgical planning of the extremity.

Intravenous contrast medium is not typically used, but in specific cases may be useful for evaluation of the vascularity of the tumor. Contrast medium should be used according to facility standards. In cases of a postarthrogram CT examination, the use of iodinated contrast medium, air, or both, may be injected into the joint capsule.

The decision to use conventional or spiral scanning is determined by the imaging facility, with consideration to the patient's ability to remain motionless during the examination. An accurate explanation of the examination process before the examination and consideration to patient comfort will reduce voluntary motion during the imaging process.

Patient Preparations

The patient is placed supine and feet first on the examination table. The patient is positioned with the midsagittal plane of the patient parallel with the longitudinal positioning light. The patient's arms should be across the abdomen or along the sides of the patient. The technologist should use positioning pads and restraining straps as needed. If the patient is supine, the placement of foam padding under the patient's knees can relieve pressure on the lower back and add to the patient's comfort, which reduces the likelihood of patient motion. Thorough but simple instructions involving the imaging procedure will also reduce patient motion. The proper placement of radiation shielding is also an essential part of every CT examination.

Imaging Protocols

AXIAL IMAGES OF THE ANKLE AND FOOT

The patient can be positioned with the legs straight and the foot perpendicular to the long axis of the table or, as an alternative, the patient can place the plantar surface flat against the examination table with the knee flexed. The first image produced can be a coronal

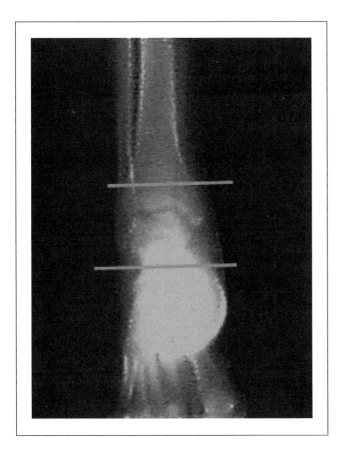

FIGURE 9-5

Anteroposterior view of the ankle to show proper centering and alignment. Lines should extend from an area superior to and through the ankle joint.

view of the ankle. From the scout image, the technologist determines whether the midsagittal plane of the patient's ankles are parallel with the long axis of the examination table. The axial slices should be perpendicular to the midsagittal plane of the ankle (Fig. 9-5).

CT EXAMINATION OF THE PELVIC GIRDLE AND HIPS

Mandatory minimum required is 5. This study must be completed on a patient, not a simulation.

Common Indications

- Evaluation of joints, bones, and soft tissues in the musculoskeletal system
- Demonstration of bone and soft tissue lesions

Imaging Considerations

A CT examination of the hips or pelvis is customized to the individual's specific clinical history. Positioning of the patient is critical; therefore, the technologist should consider symmetry of both hips at all times. Simultaneous visualization of both hips is diagnostically important for comparison. The pelvis and hips are typically scanned with the patient supine and feet first into the scanner. The patient should rotate the feet inward to position the proximal femur in the true anatomic position. A coronal scout image is used to determine the range of cross-sectional slices. The slices within the scan range should be set according to the anatomy of interest. For CT examination of the pelvis or hips, the slice thickness is a collaborative effort between the reason for the examination and the radiologist's diagnostic needs. For evaluation of small masses or fractures, thin slices will improve spatial resolution, whereas large masses can be demonstrated with thicker slices.

Imaging of musculoskeletal pelvis and hips is usually completed with the image plane being perpendicular to the region of interest. The scan FOV should be large enough to include both hips, to serve as a comparison of normal anatomy. Three-dimensional reconstructions may be helpful for surgical planning.

Intravenous contrast medium is not typically used but, in specific cases, may be useful for evaluation of the vascularity of the tumor. Contrast medium should be used per facility standards. A CT exami-

FIGURE 9-6

Anteroposterior view of the hips to show proper centering and alignment. Lines should extend from iliac crest through the symphysis pubis.

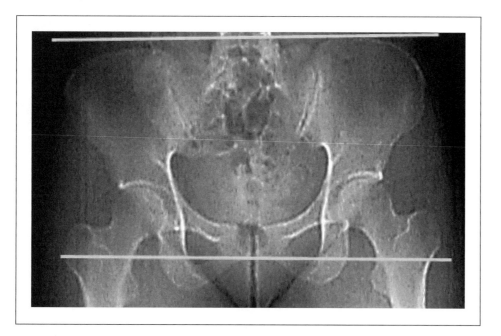

nation of joints may be completed postarthrogram. In these cases, the use of iodinated contrast medium, air, or both, may be injected into the joint capsule.

The decision to use conventional scanning or spiral scanning is determined by the imaging facility, with consideration to the patient's ability to remain motionless during the examination. An accurate explanation of the examination process before the examination and consideration to patient comfort will reduce voluntary motion during the imaging process.

Patient Preparations

The patient is placed supine and feet first on the examination table. The patient is positioned with the midsagittal plane of the patient parallel with the longitudinal positioning light. The patient's arms should be placed across the abdomen. Use positioning pads and restraining straps as needed. Taping the patient's feet together may help in symmetry and reduce motion throughout the examination. Thorough but simple instructions involving the imaging procedure will also reduce patient motion. The proper placement of radiation shielding is also an essential part of every CT examination.

Imaging Protocols

AXIAL IMAGES OF THE PELVIS OR HIPS

The first image produced is a coronal view of the pelvis, including the proximal femurs. From the scout image, the technologist determines whether the midsagittal plane of the patient is parallel with the long axis of the examination table. The axial slices should be perpendicular to the midsagittal plane. If the area of interest is the entire pelvis, the range of slices should extend from the iliac crest through the symphysis pubis. If the hip joints are the area of interest, then the range should extend through the area of interest only. The axial slices should be perpendicular to the midsagittal plane of the pelvis (Fig. 9-6).

CT MUSCULOSKELETAL EXAMINATION AFTER ARTHROGRAPHY

Elective minimum required is 3.

Common Indications

- Evaluation of synovial joints and surrounding soft tissue
- Demonstration of bone and soft tissue lesions

Imaging Considerations

An arthrogram procedure is a contrast medium study of synovial joints and demonstration of surrounding soft tissues. Arthrogram procedures are routinely performed on knees, hips, shoulder, elbow, wrist, and ankles. Arthrography of the knee and shoulder are the two most commonly performed procedures. The arthrogram procedure is routinely performed in the radiology department under the guidance of fluoroscopy. After the injection of contrast medium, the patient will be transported to the CT examination room. The CT examination after the arthrographic procedure will provide the radiologist with an axial appearance of the area of interest with enhanced visualization of the joints and surrounding muscles.

The CT examination of the affected area after an arthrographic procedure is customized to the facility's needs. The postarthrography procedure is a modified examination with images of the area of interest taken in an assortment of stages of flexion and extension. The exact postarthrography procedure is left to the discretion of the radiologist, with consideration to the specific area to be demonstrated. The technologist should be familiar with the radiologist's requirements before the examination. The slice thickness is also a collaborative effort between the reason for the examination and the radiologist's diagnostic needs. For evaluation of small masses or fractures, thin slices will improve spatial resolution, whereas large masses can be demonstrated with thicker slices.

The decision to use conventional scanning or spiral scanning is determined by the imaging facility, with consideration to the patient's ability to remain motionless during the examination. An accurate explanation of the examination process before the examination and consideration to patient comfort will reduce voluntary motion during the imaging process.

CHAPTER 10

CT Imaging Interventional Procedures

The protocols marked with asterisks must be completed on a patient, not a simulation. The protocols marked with daggers include the requirement for evaluation of laboratory values.

Procedure	Mandatory	Elective
Biopsy*†	3*†	
Drainage*†		3*†
Aspiration*†		3*†
Portography*		3*

CT INTERVENTIONAL BIOPSY PROCEDURE

Mandatory minimum required is 3. This protocol must be completed on a patient, not a simulation.

Common Indications

- Method of guidance for the biopsy of lesions in the retroperitoneum, pelvis, and mediastinum
- Demonstration of a guide needle with relationship to adjacent structures

Imaging Considerations

CT is an effective method to assist the radiologist in the performance of a biopsy procedure. A complete diagnostic CT scan is performed before the CT-guided biopsy. The principle behind a biopsy procedure is to retrieve a sample from the lesion, with a minimal amount of risk to the adjacent structures. The prebiopsy procedure will provide information for the precise entrance location of the biopsy needle. The CT examination will demonstrate the relationship of adjacent structures and the optimal entrance angulation to the area of interest. The best approach is the path that requires the least angulation and risk of puncture to adjacent structures. The technologist's role is to assist the radiologist with the patient preparation, imaging, and assessment of the site after the biopsy procedure. The patient should be informed on the process involving the biopsy and associated complications before signing the informed consent document.

LABORATORY TESTS AND VALUES

Oral contrast medium can be used to differentiate an abscess from bowel, whereas intravenous contrast medium can be used to localize an abscess and differentiate between adjacent vessels and the abscess. Contrast medium can be directly injected into cysts to reveal the true dimensions of the structure. For these reasons, it is vital to understand the laboratory tests and their associated values before any CT procedure requiring the use of contrast medium. An associated risk in a biopsy procedure is from bleeding. The risk is increased with the type and diameter of biopsy needle and with increased vascularity of the lesion. Patients with bleeding disorders may be contraindicated for a biopsy procedure, unless treatment for the disorder is completed before the biopsy. Because bleeding is a risk of any interventional procedure, the technologist should be familiar with laboratory tests evaluating the ability for the patient's blood to clot.

Before the examination, the technologist must be aware of the department standards concerning the laboratory values and consent forms concerning the injection of contrast medium and interventional procedures. Laboratory blood tests are performed to evaluate renal function before the use of intravenous contrast medium. In addition, laboratory values provide information regarding possible blood clotting disorders. These tests include prothrombin time (PT), partial thromboplastin time (PTT), platelet (thrombocyte) count, blood urea and nitrogen (BUN), and creatinine levels. The combination of these tests will influence the use of contrast medium, the continuation of the interventional procedure, or both.

PT is the laboratory test that determines the time required for the formation of clots. Prothrombin is produced by the liver and is a vitamin K–dependent glycoprotein that is necessary for the formation of a firm fibrin clot. The PT value is reported as the time required for plasma to form a clot, including the time for a laboratory control sample to clot. A value within 2 s of the control sample is considered within a normal range. The normal range for PT in a healthy adult is 10 to 15 s.

PTT is the laboratory test that evaluates the coagulation process for recalcified citrated plasma to clot after partial thromboplastin is added to it. PTT is used to monitor the effectiveness of heparin therapy and to screen for coagulation disorder. The normal adult levels of PTT is between 30 and 45 s.

Platelets are the nonnucleated cells that function for clot retraction and coagulation. Platelets are formed by the bone marrow and released into the bloodstream to function in homeostasis. Platelet (thrombocyte) count is the laboratory test for the amount of platelets present in a person's bloodstream. The normal adult level is 150,000/μL to 400,000/μL or 150 to 400 × 10^9/L.

BUN is the concentration of urea or plasma specified in terms of nitrogen content. BUN is an important indication of renal function. BUN can be elevated in disorders that can lead to renal failure. The normal range for BUN is 5 to 20 mg/dL or 1.8 to 7.1 mmol/L. The term azotemia is used in cases for which levels of urea nitrogen are elevated in the bloodstream.

Creatinine is the nitrogenous compound formed as a result of creatine metabolism. Creatinine is formed in muscle in small amounts and is passed into the bloodstream and is excreted through urine. An increased serum creatinine level is an indicator of renal dysfunction. For women, the normal creatinine level is 0.5 to 1.1 mg/dL or 47 to 97 μmol/L. The creatinine level for men is slightly higher, i.e., the normal level for the adult male is 0.6 to 1.2 mg/dL or 53 to 106 μmol/L.

Preimaging Considerations and Patient Preparations

The preimaging preparations are determined by the contrast manufacturer and radiologist preference. The specific protocol may vary between individual imaging facilities; therefore, the technologist should be aware of specific protocols for the imaging facility. The evening before the biopsy procedure, the patient is typically instructed to have a clear liquid diet. The patient should remain NPO after midnight if the biopsy is completed the following morning. The technologist should inform the patient of precautions involving contrast medium and acquire all necessary consent forms before beginning the examination. The technologist should prepare the necessary equipment within the scan room. The use of a standard biopsy tray will often include the items listed in Table 10-1. Any item specific to

TABLE 10-1

Items Contained Within a Sterile Biopsy or Aspiration and Drainage Tray

25G × ⅝ in. needle	0.9% Sodium chloride, 5 mL
21G × 1½ in. needle	3 × 3 Gauze (6)
18G Blunt needle	Fenestrated drape
Needle stop	Plastic ruler
Alcohol wipe	Towel, 18 × 26 in.
5-mL LL syringe	Drape, 24 × 36 in.
10-mL LL syringe	Band-Aid
No. 11 Scalpel assembly	Slides, frosted end (8)
PVP swabsticks	Needle counter
1% Xylocaine, 5 mL	Sterile indicator
Solution cup	

the radiologist's needs should be included in the list of preparations of the biopsy tray. These items will include the radiologist's choice of catheters, dilators, guide wires, and biopsy needles.

If there are previous CT films concerning the area of interest, the technologist should review the films and have them ready for viewing by the radiologist. The patient's position is dependent on the area of interest and the location that the biopsy needle is to enter. Before the procedure, the patient should be instructed for the proper breathing techniques. Normally, the patient will hold his or her breath during the actual biopsy process. After insertion of the biopsy needle, the patient is instructed to breathe quietly and consistently.

Imaging Protocols

The actual biopsy process is dictated by the imaging facility. The technologist should be aware of the specifics of the facility before assisting the radiologist with the biopsy procedure.

A scout image of the patient is attained, and a scan range through the area of interest is determined. The most direct approach requiring the least amount of angulation and risk to adjacent tissues is the ideal location for the entrance of the biopsy needle. After location of the lesion, the radiologist will select an entrance site and place a metallic marker over the site. The use of geometric measurements may be necessary to locate the distance between the lesion and the tissue surface. The technologist should save images concerning the area of interest. These images will include the entire area of interest, from the superior to inferior borders. After the site is selected, the technologist will take serial images through the area of interest when instructed by the radiologist.

The technologist will prepare the site according to aseptic guidelines. The area of interest is draped according to the radiologist's preference. The radiologist will administer a local anesthetic, then insert the guide needle into the area of interest. At this time, the technologist will scan the site to assess the location of the guide needle. The needle will have a hyperintense (bright) appearance on the image. There will be shadowing inferior to the needle tip. Some facilities use a lateral scout image to correlate the location of the needle tip. All images demonstrating needle placement into the area of interest should be saved.

During and after the biopsy, the technologist will scan the area of interest for evaluation. Upon completion of the procedure, the radiologist and technologist will review the CT images. The technologist now assists the radiologist in the process of dressing the biopsy entrance location. Part of the postprocedural duties of the technologist include monitoring and recording of vital signs. Postprocedural CT images or radiographic films are completed to evaluate for complications such as hemothorax or pneumothorax. Patients are typically kept for an observation period of 1 to 2 h. The technologist should inform the patient of any additional instructions and release the patient upon the approval of the radiologist.

CT INTERVENTIONAL DRAINAGE PROCEDURE

Elective minimum required is 3. This protocol must be completed on a patient, not a simulation.

Common Indications

- Method of guidance for the drainage of an abscess within the retroperitoneum, pelvis, and mediastinum
- Demonstration of relationship of adjacent structures before needle placement

Imaging Considerations

The purpose of an abscess drainage is for the removal of fluid and simultaneously avoiding the perforation to adjacent structures. Computed tomography is an effective method to assist the radiologist in the performance of a drainage procedure. This procedure will provide the information for precise entrance location of the drainage catheter. The CT examination demonstrates the relationship of adjacent structures and the optimal entrance angulation to the area of interest. The optimal approach will require the least angulation and risk of puncture to adjacent structure. The technologist's role is to assist the radiologist through the drainage procedure. The patient should be informed on the process involving the procedure and associated complications before signing the informed consent document.

LABORATORY TESTS AND VALUE

Oral contrast medium can be used to differentiate an abscess from bowel, whereas intravenous contrast medium can be used to localize an abscess and differentiate between adjacent vessels and the abscess. After drainage of an abscess, contrast medium can be injected into the abscess cavity to demonstrate any undrained loculated portions of the abscess and to outline fistulous tracts. For these reasons, it is vital to understand the laboratory tests and their associated values before any CT procedure requiring the use of contrast medium. Because bleeding is a risk of any interventional procedure, the technologist should be familiar with laboratory tests evaluating the ability for the patient's blood to clot.

Before the examination, the technologist must be aware of the department standards concerning the laboratory values and consent forms concerning the injection of contrast medium and interventional procedures. Laboratory blood tests are performed to evaluate renal function before the use of intravenous contrast medium. In addition, laboratory values provide information regarding possible blood clotting disorders. These laboratory tests include PT, PTT, platelet (thrombocyte) count, BUN, and creatinine levels. The combination of

115

these tests will influence the use of contrast medium, the continuation of the interventional procedure, or both.

PT is the laboratory test that determines the time required for the formation of clots. Prothrombin is produced by the liver and is a vitamin K–dependent glycoprotein that is necessary for the formation of a firm fibrin clot. The PT value is reported as the time required for plasma to form a clot, including the time for a laboratory control sample to clot. A value within 2 s of the control sample is considered within a normal range. The normal range for PT in a healthy adult is 10 to 15 s.

PTT is the laboratory test that evaluates the coagulation process for recalcified citrated plasma to clot after partial thromboplastin is added to it. PTT is used to monitor the effectiveness of heparin therapy and to screen for coagulation disorder. The normal adult levels of PTT is between 30 and 45 s.

Platelets are the nonnucleated cells that function for clot retraction and coagulation. Platelets are formed by the bone marrow and released into the bloodstream to function in homeostasis. Platelet (thrombocyte) count is the laboratory test for the amount of platelets present in a person's bloodstream. The normal adult level is $150,000/\mu L$ to $400,000/\mu L$ or 150 to $400 \times 10^9/L$.

BUN is the concentration of urea or plasma specified in terms of nitrogen content. BUN is an important indication of renal function. BUN can be elevated in disorders that can lead to renal failure. The normal range for BUN is 5 to 20 mg/dL or 1.8 to 7.1 mmol/L. The term azotemia is used in cases for which levels of urea nitrogen are elevated in the bloodstream.

Creatinine is the nitrogenous compound formed as a result of creatine metabolism. Creatinine is formed in muscle in small amounts and is passed into the bloodstream and is excreted through urine. An increased serum creatinine level is an indicator of renal dysfunction. For women, the normal creatinine level is 0.5 to 1.1 mg/dL or 47 to 97 μmol/L. The creatinine level for men is slightly higher, i.e., the level for adult males is 0.6 to 1.2 mg/dL or 53 to 106 μmol/L.

Preimaging Considerations and Patient Preparations

The preimaging preparations are determined by the contrast manufacturer and the radiologist's preference. The specific protocol may vary between individual imaging facilities; therefore, the technologist should be aware of specific protocols for the imaging facility. The evening before the drainage procedure, the patient is typically instructed to have a clear liquid diet. The patient should remain NPO after midnight if the procedure is to be completed the following morning. The technologist should inform the patient of precautions involving contrast medium and acquire all necessary consent forms before beginning the examination. The technologist should prepare the necessary equipment within the scan room. The use of a standard drainage kit will often include the items listed in Table 10-2. Any item

TABLE 10-2

Items Contained Within a Sterile Aspiration and Drainage Tray

25G × ⅝ in. needle	0.9% Sodium chloride, 5 mL
21G × 1½ in. needle	3 × 3 Gauze (6)
18G Blunt needle	Fenestrated drape
Needle stop	Plastic ruler
Alcohol wipe	Towel, 18 × 26 in.
5-mL LL syringe	Drape, 24 × 36 in.
10-mL LL syringe	Band-Aid
No. 11 Scalpel assembly	Specimen tubes (3)
PVP swabsticks	Needle counter
1% Xylocaine, 5 mL	Sterile indicator
Solution cup	

specific to the radiologist's needs should be included in the list of preparations of the drainage kit. These items will include the radiologist's choice of catheters, dilators, guide wires, and needles.

If there are previous CT films concerning the area of interest, the technologist should review the films and have them ready for viewing by the radiologist. The patient's position is dependent on the area of interest and the location where the needle is to enter. Before the procedure, the patient should be instructed for the proper breathing instruction. Typically, the patient will hold his or her breath during the actual insertion of the needle. After insertion of the needle, the patient is instructed to breathe quietly and consistently.

Imaging Protocols

The actual drainage process is dictated by the imaging facility. The technologist should be aware of the specifics of the facility before assisting the radiologist with the drainage procedure. A scout image of the patient is attained, and a scan range through the area of interest is determined. The most direct approach requiring the least amount of angulation and risk to adjacent tissues is the ideal entrance site for the guide needle. After the abscess is located, the radiologist will select an entrance site and place a radiopaque marker over the site. The use of geometric measurements may be necessary to locate the distance between the abscess and the tissue surface. The technologist should save the images concerning the area of interest. These images will include the entire area of interest, from the superior to inferior borders. After the site is selected, the technologist will take serial images through the area of interest when instructed by the radiologist. The center of the abscess is the optimal site for the entrance of the drainage needle.

The technologist will prepare the site according to aseptic guidelines and drape the area according to the radiologist's preference. The radiologist will administer a local anesthetic, then insert the guide needle into the area of interest. At this time, the technologist will scan the site to assess the location of the guide needle. The needle will have a hyperintense (bright) appearance on the image. There will be shadowing inferior to the needle tip. Some facilities use a lateral scout image to correlate the location of the needle tip. The technologist should save the image showing needle placement into the area of interest.

The technologist will assist the radiologist in the process of the fluid sampling. The specimen tubes should be labeled with the proper patient information. The radiologist will try and aspirate a fluid sample. If this is not successful, the radiologist may use a drainage catheter. All fluid should not be removed at this time if a drainage tube is considered. After proper placement of the drainage tube, the radiologist will secure the end with tape or suture. The cavity is now aspirated until dry and flushed with normal saline until clear. Water soluble contrast medium may be injected into the abscess cavity to demonstrate any undrained loculated portions of the abscess and to outline fistulous tracts. The drainage tube can be left from 4 to 7 days, or until the drainage has reduced. The drainage catheter is typically removed or replaced under fluoroscopic monitoring. During and after the drainage, the technologist will scan the area of interest for evaluation. Upon completion of the procedure, the radiologist and technologist review the CT images. Postprocedural CT images or radiographic films are completed to evaluate for complications such as hemothorax or pneumothorax. Part of the postprocedural duties of the technologist include monitoring and recording of vital signs. The technologist should inform the patient of any additional instructions and release the patient upon the approval of the radiologist.

CT INTERVENTIONAL ASPIRATION PROCEDURE

Elective minimum required is 3. This protocol must be completed on a patient, not a simulation.

Common Indications

- Method of guidance for the cytology aspiration in areas of the retroperitoneum, pelvis, and mediastinum
- Demonstration of relationship of adjacent structures before needle placement

Imaging Considerations

The purpose of an aspiration is for the removal of material for cytologic examination, while simultaneously avoiding the perforation to adjacent structures. Computed tomography is an effective method to assist the radiologist in the performance of an aspiration procedure. The CT procedure will provide the information for precise entrance location of the aspiration needle. The CT examination demonstrates the relationship of adjacent structures and the optimal entrance angulation and distance to the area of interest. The optimal approach will require the least angulation and risk of puncture to adjacent structure. The technologist's role is to assist the radiologist through the aspiration procedure. The patient should be informed on the process involving the aspiration and associated complications before signing the informed consent document.

There are a variety of fine-gauge needles used for aspiration purposes. There are advantages and disadvantages of each type. In addition, the technologist should be aware of the physician's preference for the type and usage of each needle. Normally a 21- to 22-gauge needle is used for aspirations. The use of a larger gauge needle will allow for more blood, but little additional cytologic material.

LABORATORY TESTS AND VALUE

Oral contrast medium can be used to differentiate an abscess from bowel, whereas intravenous contrast medium can be used to localize an abscess and differentiate between adjacent vessels and the abscess. For these reasons, it is vital to understand the laboratory tests and their associated values before any CT procedure requiring the use of contrast medium. Bleeding is a risk of any interventional procedure; because of this, the technologist should be familiar with laboratory tests evaluating the ability of the patient's blood to clot. The patient should be informed on the process involving the procedure and associated complications before signing the informed consent document.

Before the examination, the technologist must be aware of the department standards concerning the laboratory values and consent forms concerning the injection of contrast medium and interventional procedures. Laboratory blood tests are performed to evaluate renal function before the use of intravenous contrast medium. In addition, laboratory values provide information regarding possible blood clotting disorders. These laboratory tests include PT, PTT, platelet (thrombocyte) count, BUN, and creatinine levels. The combination of these tests will influence the use of contrast medium, the continuation of the interventional procedure, or both.

PT is the laboratory test that determines the time required for the formation of clots. Prothrombin is produced by the liver and is a vitamin K–dependent glycoprotein that is necessary for the formation of a firm fibrin clot. The PT value is reported as the time required for plasma to form a clot, including the time for a laboratory control sample to clot. A value within 2 s of the control sample is considered

119

within a normal range. The normal range for PT in a healthy adult is 10 to 15 s.

PTT is the laboratory test that evaluates the coagulation process for recalcified citrated plasma to clot after partial thromboplastin is added to it. PTT is used to monitor the effectiveness of heparin therapy and to screen for coagulation disorder. The normal adult levels of PTT is between 30 and 45 s.

Platelets are the nonnucleated cells that function for clot retraction and coagulation. Platelets are formed by the bone marrow and released into the bloodstream to function in homeostasis. Platelet (thrombocyte) count is the laboratory test for the amount of platelets present in a person's bloodstream. The normal adult level is 150,000/μL to 400,000/μL or 150 to 400 × 10^9/L.

BUN is the concentration of urea or plasma specified in terms of nitrogen content. BUN is an important indication of renal function. BUN can be elevated in disorders that can lead to renal failure. The normal range for BUN is 5 to 20 mg/dL or 1.8 to 7.1 mmol/L. The term azotemia is used in cases for which levels of urea nitrogen are elevated in the bloodstream.

Creatinine is the nitrogenous compound formed as a result of creatine metabolism. Creatinine is formed in muscle in small amounts and is passed into the bloodstream and is excreted through urine. An increased serum creatinine level is an indicator of renal dysfunction. For women, the normal creatinine level is 0.5 to 1.1 mg/dL or 47 to 97 μmol/L. The creatinine level for men is slightly higher, i.e., the normal level for adult males is 0.6 to 1.2 mg/dL or 53 to 106 μmol/L.

Preimaging Considerations and Patient Preparations

The preimaging preparations are determined by the contrast manufacturer and the radiologist's preference. The specific protocol may vary between individual imaging facilities; therefore, the technologist should be aware of specific protocols for the imaging facility. The evening before the aspiration procedure, the patient is typically instructed to have a clear liquid diet. The patient should remain NPO after midnight if the procedure is to be completed the following morning. The technologist should prepare the necessary equipment within the scan room. The use of a standard aspiration kit will often include the items listed in Table 10-3. Any item specific to the radiologist's needs should be included in the list of preparations. These items will include the radiologist's choice of catheters, dilators, guide wires, and needles.

If there are previous CT films concerning the area of interest, the technologist should review the films and have them ready for viewing by the radiologist. The patient's position is dependent on the area of interest and the location that the needle is to enter. Before the procedure, the patient should be instructed for the proper breathing techniques. Typically, the patient will hold his or her breath during the

TABLE 10-3

Items Contained Within a Sterile Aspiration and Drainage Tray

25G × ⅝ in. needle	0.9% Sodium chloride, 5 mL
21G × 1½ in. needle	3 × 3 Gauze (6)
18G Blunt needle	Fenestrated drape
Needle stop	Plastic ruler
Alcohol wipe	Towel, 18 × 26 in.
5-mL LL syringe	Drape, 24 × 36 in.
10-mL LL syringe	Band-Aid
No. 11 Scalpel assembly	Specimen tubes (3)
PVP swabsticks	Needle counter
1% Xylocaine, 5 mL	Sterile indicator
Solution cup	

actual insertion of the needle. After insertion of the needle, the patient is instructed to breathe quietly and consistently.

Imaging Protocols

The actual aspiration process is dictated by the imaging facility. The technologist should be aware of the specifics of the facility before assisting the radiologist with the drainage procedure. A scout image of the patient is attained, and a scan range through the area of interest is determined. The most direct approach requiring the least amount of angulation and risk to adjacent tissues is the ideal entrance site for the guide needle. After the abscess is located, the radiologist will select an entrance site and place a radiopaque marker over the site. The use of geometric measurements may be necessary to locate the distance between the abscess and the tissue surface. The technologist should save the images concerning the area of interest. These images will include the entire area of interest, from the superior to inferior borders. After the site is selected, the technologist will take serial images through the area of interest when instructed by the radiologist.

The technologist will prepare the site according to aseptic guidelines and drape the area according to the radiologist's preference. The radiologist will administer a local anesthetic, then insert the needle into the area of interest. At this time, the technologist will scan the site to assess the location of the needle. The needle will have a hyperintense (bright) appearance on the image. There will be shadowing inferior to the needle tip. Some facilities use a lateral scout image to correlate the location of the needle tip. The technologist should save the image showing needle placement into the area of interest.

The technologist will assist the radiologist in the process of the fluid sampling. The specimen containers should be labeled with the proper patient information. The radiologist will try and aspirate a fluid sample. During and after the aspiration procedure, the technologist will scan the area of interest for evaluation. Upon completion of the procedure, the radiologist and technologist review the CT images. Postprocedural CT images or radiographic films are completed to evaluate for complications such as hemothorax or pneumothorax. Part of the postprocedural duties of the technologist include monitoring and recording of vital signs. The technologist should inform the patient of any additional instructions and release the patient upon the approval of the radiologist.

CT INTERVENTIONAL PORTOGRAPHY PROCEDURE

Elective minimum required is 3. This protocol must be completed on a patient, not a simulation.

Common Indications

- Preoperative evaluation for the location and number of metastatic lesions in the area of the liver for accurate surgical planning

Imaging Considerations

Computed tomography with arterial portography (CTAP) is the process of introducing contrast medium into the portal venous blood supply by means of the superior mesenteric artery. This method of injection prevents the dilution of the contrast medium by the normal circulatory process. Because of the increased speed, spiral computed tomography is the ideal process for scanning after the injection of contrast medium into the portal venous system. All necessary consent and contrast medium precautions must be taken with CTAP as with any interventional examination. The process of CTAP begins in the angiography suite, where a celiac, superior mesenteric artery (SMA) angiography is performed to evaluate any variant anatomy to the celiac or SMA. The catheter placed in the patient's SMA will allow for the circulation of contrast medium from the colon into the liver. The type and amount of contrast will vary among institutions. The amount up to 150 mL at a rate of 1.5 mL/s of iodinated contrast agent is typical for CTAP (Fishman and Jeffrey, 1995). The method of direct injection into the area of interest or organ of interest provides a more specific examination instead of the injection of contrast medium into the blood circulatory system. The process of CTAP, used for lesion localization, has a reported sensitivity of 81 to 91% (Fishman and Jeffrey, 1995).

A noncontrasted study of the liver is performed for location and comparison of the liver tissue before the injection of contrast medium. The technologist then repositions the patient to locate the liver. The patient is again informed of the proper breath-holding sequence. After the injection of contrast medium and the designated delay time, the technologist begins to scan the contrasted portion of the CTAP. The images are reconstructed according to the radiologist's preferences.

Lesions within the liver do not enhance at the same rate as normal liver tissue. Vascular lesions of the liver are usually supplied by the hepatic arteries; therefore, lesions that are highly vascular will enhance faster than normal liver tissue. Lesions of the liver that have poor vascularity will enhance slower than the normal liver tissue. For these reasons, it is important for the technologist to understand the optimal delay between injection of contrast medium and the liver tissue and lesion becoming isodense. Spiral scanning and rapid scanning techniques have improved the specificity of lesion detection in computed tomography. Spiral computed tomography has enabled the technologist to scan the entire liver in under 30 s. This allows for reduction in motion artifacts and slice misregistration, because the patient normally can hold his or her breath through the entire acquisition of image data.

CHAPTER 11

CT Special Procedures

The protocols marked with asterisks must be completed on a patient, not a simulation.

Procedure	Mandatory	Elective
Leg length*		3*
Pelvimetry*		3*
Radiation therapy planning*		3*
Spiral*		5*
Stereotaxis*		3*
Pediatric imaging* (6 years or under)		5*
Nonincremental dynamic scanning		3
Multiplanar reconstruction (postprocessing only)	5	
3D Vascular reconstruction (postprocessing only)		5
3D Bone reconstruction (postprocessing only)		5
Virtual reality* (Fly Through, Navigator) (including postprocessing)		3*

CT SPECIAL PROCEDURES FOR STUDIES OF LEG LENGTH

Elective minimum required is 3. This protocol must be completed on a patient, not a simulation.

Common Indications

- Accurate assessment of leg length discrepancy
- Assessment of rotational deformities of long bones that cause problems in gait
- Assessment of tibial torsion, femoral anteversion, or acetabular anteversion

Imaging Considerations

The advantages of performing leg length evaluation studies by using computed tomography include speed and accuracy. Although the dosage for the overall examination is less with the use of computed tomography (Seeram, 1994), the technologist must be aware of radiation protection. The patient should be shielded from radiation originating from the anterior, posterior, and lateral directions. In addition, the strategic placement of gonadal shielding is necessary. Leg length studies routinely are completed on adolescent patients. Therefore, consideration to reducing the mAs to accommodate the size difference will also reduce the patient dose. The patient normally does not require any additional pre-examination preparation for the CT leg length study.

Before imaging, it is important for the technologist to view previous films and have them available for viewing by the radiologist. This process also assures the patient that the CT study is the optimal examination for the patient's needs. Before placing the patient on the examination table, the technologist should explain the process to both the patient and the adults accompanying the patient. The time taken to explain the process will be returned with cooperation and reduction of motion artifacts in the resulting images.

The patient is positioned supine and feet first into the gantry. The patient's arms should be placed out of the field of view to avoid artifacts and unnecessary exposure. The technologist must align the patient to the center of the gantry table. Additional positioning padding and restraining devices may be necessary. The table is raised to the level where the midcoronal plane of the legs intersects the horizontal positioning light. The technologist will take a scout image extending from hip joints through knee joints. A second scout may be necessary to include the range from knee joints through ankle joints. Before allowing the patient to leave the examination table, it is recommended that the images be viewed by the radiologist to avoid rescheduling for another CT examination. The measurement for leg lengths can be completed with the assistance of the electronic measuring feature available in the CT software. Filming is completed according to the radiologist's preference.

CT SPECIAL PROCEDURES FOR PELVIMETRY

Elective minimum required is 3. This protocol must be completed on a patient, not a simulation.

Common Indications

- Evaluation for pelvic inadequacy
- Predelivery identification of a hyperextended fetal head

• Whenever a vaginal delivery is being considered for a patient with a fetal breech presentation

Imaging Considerations

According to Moss, Gamsu, and Genant (1992), the amount of radiation the fetus receives throughout the pelvimetry examination process is considerably less using computed tomography compared with conventional radiography. This occurs because there is seldom a repeat study because of the patient's size and density compared with a typical radiograph. For these reasons, the use of CT pelvimetry including a single slice has replaced the use of conventional radiography. The CT pelvimetry study is typically completed with a reduction in the mAs to further reduce the radiation exposure to the patient and fetus. The patient normally does not require any additional pre-examination preparation for the CT pelvimetry study.

The technologist should have all imaging parameters set before positioning the patient. This will reduce the time required for the patient to remain in a supine and motion-free position. The patient is positioned supine and head first into the gantry opening. The patient should place her arms above her head to reduce exposure and artifacts entering the field of view. The patient is positioned to the center of the gantry table. The coronal scout image should extend from the iliac crest through the symphysis pubis. A lateral scout image will

FIGURE 11-1

Coronal scout of pelvis showing measurement of transverse pelvis (for pelvimetry).

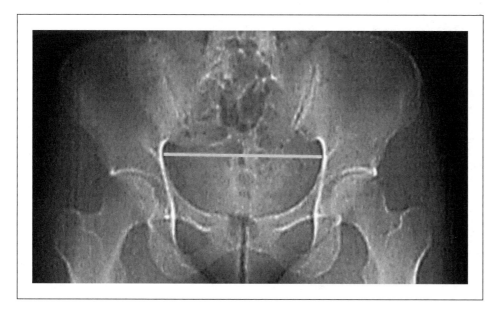

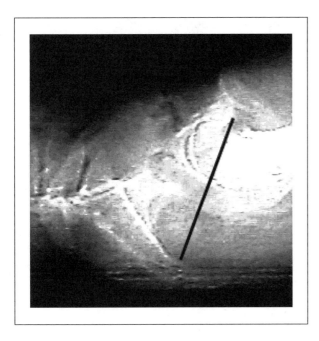

FIGURE 11-2

Lateral scout of pelvis showing measurement of anteroposterior dimension of the pelvic inlet extending from the symphysis to the sacral prominence (for pelvimetry).

then extend from the sacral promontory to the upper portion of the symphysis pubis. Typically a single axial image will be selected at the level of the fovea of the femoral heads (Figs. 11-1 and 11-2).

FIGURE 11-3

Axial slice through the fovea of the femoral heads. Measurement extending from the ischial spines (for pelvimetry).

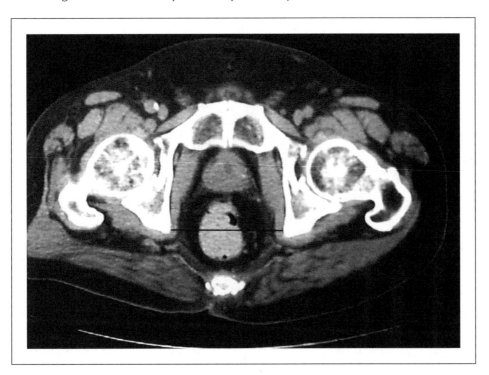

The measurements are completed with the electronic calipers software. The coronal scout will permit the measurement of the widest point of the transverse diameter of the pelvis (normal, >12.0 cm). The lateral scout image is used to measure the pelvic inlet or true conjugate. This measurement is from the sacral promontory to the upper portion of the symphysis pubis (normal, >11 cm). The final measurement is determined at the level of the fovea of the femoral heads. This is the interspinous distance between the two points connecting the ischial spines at the level of the fovea of the femoral heads. This measurements is normally greater than 10 cm (Fig. 11-3).

CT SPECIAL PROCEDURES FOR RADIATION THERAPY PLANNING

Elective minimum required is 3. This protocol must be completed on a patient, not a simulation.

Common Indications

- Calculation of physical location and electron densities of tissues for dose computations used in radiation treatment planning

Imaging Considerations

CT examinations completed for the preparation of radiation therapy planning is a collaborative effort of the radiology and radiation oncology departments. Before radiation therapy, patients may be examined by conventional computed tomography. The positioning of the patient is dependent on the position for treating the designated area. The patient should be positioned exactly as he or she will receive the radiation treatments. Depending on departmental procedures, the technologist may be required to take measurements of tumors. In addition, the technologist may be asked to demonstrate the density of the tumor by using Hounsfield units within the area of interest.

The images are filmed in a manner similar to that for a traditional CT examination for the specific anatomic part. After the examination, the processed data is stored on a separate magnetic tape or disc. The radiation oncology department will use the disc information in the planning for radiation therapy. The images on disc and films are used to determine the size, shape, and density of the area of interest. In addition, the CT images will provide information concerning adjacent structures to the treatment site. The images will be used to determine the optimal angle of entrance and proper dosage. In many cases, after radiation therapy, the patient will again receive a follow-up CT examination to track and determine the success of the treatment. This follow-up examination will include evaluation to structures adjacent to the treatment site.

CT SPECIAL PROCEDURES FOR SPIRAL IMAGING

Elective minimum required is 5. This protocol must be completed on a patient, not a simulation.

Common Indications

- Faster scanning through the area of interest
- Reduction in slice misregistration
- Reduction in voluntary motion artifacts

Imaging Considerations

Spiral imaging is a topic worthy of an entire book. It is not the purpose of this manual to discuss the fine points and technicalities of spiral imaging; therefore, the discussion will be in general terms. However, I would advise all practicing CT technologists to investigate in detail the physical principles involved in spiral imaging because of its current widespread use.

Spiral imaging became available through the development of the slip ring technology. Before slip ring technology, the x-ray tube of the CT scanner could rotate in one direction and not beyond one revolution. Upon completion of the revolution, the x-ray tube had to reverse directions to avoid wrapping of the electrical cables that supply the power to the components within the gantry unit. Slip ring technology is similar to a model race car set. The electricity to the electrical motors within the model cars is carried through the metal strips embedded into the plastic race track. This simple analogy explains the principle of slip ring technology. The ring stays in a stationary position while the x-ray tube rotates around the perimeter. In addition to the slip ring technology, it became necessary to develop an x-ray tube with higher heat and load capacities.

The process is referred to as "spiral or helical" imaging because of the shape of the resulting information. Conventional CT imaging is a repetitious process of the tube rotation and table movement. Upon completion of the rotation, the patient is advanced into the gantry opening the distance equal to the designated slice thickness. The process is repeated through the entire area of interest. The information gathered from this process is from a true planar reference. Interscan delay is a delay time from the beginning of the tube rotation until the next tube rotation. The interscan delay includes the scan time and the time it takes the table to advance to the next location.

With spiral scanning, the x-ray tube rotates on the slip ring tract. During the rotation, the tube can generate a constant flow of x-rays. Because the table is in constant motion, and simultaneous with the rotation of the x-ray tube, the information gathered is not planar, but instead in the shape of a spiral. The relationship between the rotation of the x-ray tube and the slice thickness is termed "pitch." To an extent the technologist can determine the pitch of machine. A pitch of 1:1 means that the table advances the equal distance to the selected slice thickness per rotation of the tube. A pitch of 2:1 means that the table advances twice as far as the selected slice thickness per rotation. The higher the value of pitch, the less planar the information gathered. The analogy of stretching a spring longer is similar to increasing the pitch of the CT scanner.

The advantages of spiral CT scanning include speed, reduction in slice misregistration, reduced amounts of intravenous contrast medium, and improvement of 3D and multiplanar reconstructions. Spiral computed tomography is used in many forms of imaging. The use of spiral computed tomography for imaging of the head, chest, abdomen, and pelvis is common practice. Anytime there is a need for reconstruction of information into a 3D or multiplanar image, the use of spiral data acquisition is the optimal choice.

Conventional scanning typically takes a matter of minutes to scan through the patient's abdomen. Scan times for spiral imaging can now be reduced to a matter of seconds to cover the same anatomic distance. If the technologist is performing an abdomen-pelvis examination after the intravenous contrast injection, it is now possible to complete the entire distance before the contrast medium has had sufficient time to reach the pelvis. The technologist needs to be aware of postinjection delay times before working with imaging procedures requiring the use of injectable contrast medium.

CT SPECIAL PROCEDURES FOR STEREOTACTIC SURGICAL PLANNING

Elective minimum required is 3. This protocol must be completed on a patient, not a simulation.

Common Indications

- Exact localization for the biopsy of intracranial lesions
- Aspiration of brain abscess or cystic structures
- Functional neurosurgery

Imaging Considerations

The purchase of the stereotactic device and appropriate software is necessary before performing this procedure. The protocols used are determined by the manufacturer of the stereotactic device and software. The patient's head is placed in the stereotactic device and secured to ensure complete immobilization. The stereotactic device and software is used to localize the area of interest in all three dimensions. The horizontal dimension is referred to as the x axis. The x axis will extend from the patient's left to right lateral margins. The technologist can determine the distance from the area of interest to the center of the x axis with assistance of the stereotactic software. The y axis extends from the anterior to posterior dimensions of the patient's head. Again, the stereotactic software will enable the technologist to determine the location from the center of the y axis to the area of interest. The superior to inferior dimension of the patient is referred to as the z axis. The location of the tumor in the z axis can be localized by the table position. The CT examination is completed through the area of interest.

After the area of interest is located, the table position is noted. The table is then returned to the location of the area of interest. The x and y axes are determined and adjustments made to the stereotactic device according to manufacturer's specifications. After the adjustments, the stereotactic device is locked into position in both the x and y axes. The purpose of localization is to provide the physician with entrance to the area of interest from multiple angles of the skull. To provide the exact localization to the area of interest, the technologist must be aware of volume imaging and spatial resolution. To provide the optimal spatial resolution and reduce volume imaging, the technologist should use a thin slice thickness through the area of interest. In addition, the technologist should use the appropriate field of view when imaging. It has been determined that a slice thickness of 1.5 mm and a field of view of 25 cm has yielded accuracy of 0.3 mm in the x and y axes and 0.6 mm in the z axis. The combination of these three techniques will improve the spatial resolution and accuracy of the stereotactic procedure.

CT SPECIAL PROCEDURES FOR PEDIATRIC IMAGING (6 YEARS OR YOUNGER)

Elective minimum required is 5. This protocol must be completed on a patient, not a simulation.

Common Indications

- Assessment of head trauma, acute hemorrhage, and the detection of calcification
- Assessment of brain tumors
- Evaluation of disk protrusion

Imaging Considerations

The goals of pediatric CT imaging include acquiring the best image in the shortest possible time, with the least amount of discomfort to the patient. The success of this process can be determined by the amount of preparation completed before the patient enters the imaging room.

The technologist should review the patient's previous films and medical history. The preview of history and films discussed with the radiologist will verify if the CT examination is the proper choice. Magnetic resonance imaging has become the examination of choice for pediatric patients concerning studies of the central nervous system. If intravenous contrast medium is required for the examination, it should be prepared before the arrival of the patient into the examination room. The amount and method of administration of contrast medium is determined according to department standards and radiologist preference.

An important rule in pediatric imagining is never to lie to the patient or parents. At the same time, it is best to be specific but not necessarily technical about the examination. Parents should have an understanding about the examination process and the length of time necessary to complete the examination. A thorough explanation before the examination will reduce anxiety and improve the assistance by both parent and child. When scheduling young patients, the child should be encouraged to bring his or her favorite blanket or stuffed animal.

If sedation is determined necessary for patients between 3 months and 5 years of age, it should be prepared before the examination. Sedation of the pediatric patient is a collaborative effort between the anesthesiologist and radiologist. The proper protocol involving sedation of pediatric patients should be clearly understood by the CT technologist before examinations. Ideally, the patient should have an intravenous site established before entering the scan room if the use of injectable contrast medium is to be used. Nonionic contrast medium has reduced the amount of reactions after the injection. However, this does *not* relieve the technologist from acquiring a complete patient history before the examination. Physical visualization of the injection site is a necessary precaution every technologist should take with pediatric patients.

Radiation protection is another item the technologist is responsible for before imaging the pediatric patient. As with every patient being examined by computed tomography, the shielding must protect the patient from the surrounding x-ray pattern. When possible, the technologist should lay shielding on the examination table before the arrival of the patient. Patients should be shielded from above and below, while avoiding shielding the area of interest. For imaging neonatal patients, it is recommended to wrap a warm blanket around the patient before applying shielding. This process reduces neonate movement and provides a relaxing atmosphere. If the parent must accompany the patient through the examination, it is the responsibility of the technologist to provide necessary shielding and place the parent in a safe location.

With consideration to the patient's size and growth maturity, the response is to reduce the technical factors during the scanning process. It is important not to reduce the technical factors so much that there will be a loss to image quality. Patient positioning also requires alterations when compared with adult-sized patients. The pediatric patient may require additional positioning sponges and restraining devices to ensure centering to the gantry and immobilization. It is the responsibility of the technologist to be familiar with pediatric protocols before the examination. Scan protocols for pediatrics will typically change slice thickness; scan with large gaps between the slices to reduce radiation dose.

CT SPECIAL PROCEDURES FOR NONINCREMENTAL DYNAMIC SCANNING

Elective minimum required is 3.

Common Indications

- The visualization of the effect for a bolus contrast injection to a specific anatomic site or lesion
- Diagnosis of liver hemangiomas
- Evaluation of dissection within the aorta

Imaging Considerations

Dynamic scanning is a process of rapid image acquisition, rapid in terms of faster than normal conventional scanning. This process is accomplished by reducing the mAs to reduce the rapid buildup of heat during image acquisition. Dynamic nonincremental scanning is typically applied to areas of the liver and aorta. The principle of nonincremental dynamic scanning is to allow the technologist to gather images through the area of interest. During this process, intravenous contrast medium is injected and the enhancement of the area of interest is scanned while the contrast enhancement changes though the various stages of enhancement. The process of rapid image acquisition allows the technologist to attain multiple images while the patient maintains a single breath hold.

In the youth of computed tomography, the term *dynamic* meant that it was a scanning method faster than the normal scan process. With the recent improvement of slip ring technology and higher heat capacity of x-ray tubes, the new CT scanner can now perform faster than the older scanners during the "dynamic" era. This is why the current term has changed to *rapid acquisition scanning* or *rapid scan*.

The intravenous injection site is prepared before the initial scanning process. The scanning procedure for the nonincremental rapid scan begins with the noncontrast portion of the CT examination. The area of interest is selected from the acquired noncontrasted images. The technologist should change the image annotation to read "contrast" before the injection. The examination table is repositioned to the area of interest. The scanning process begins after the injection of the contrast medium. The success of this procedure is dependent on the preparations of the technologist. After the image acquisition, the technologist and radiologist should view the images before dismissing the patient.

CT SPECIAL PROCEDURES FOR MULTIPLANAR RECONSTRUCTION (POSTPROCESSING ONLY)

Mandatory minimum required is 5.

Common Indications

- The visualization of existing images into a different imaging plane
- The demonstration of specific anatomy in relation to the surrounding structures
- For the determination of the extent of lesions or fractures
- The localization of intraarticular bone fragments or foreign bodies

Imaging Considerations

Multiplanar reconstruction (MPR) is a process of taking the acquired information and reconstructing it for display in another plane. Unlike the appearance of 3D images, MPR has the appearance of a slice of information in different imaging planes such as obliquities and true planar displays. Some software packages allow for the re-formation of information of two imaging planes simultaneously. This creates an image with a curved appearance. The MPR software reconstruction process consists of taking the acquired images and stacking them together as if it were a volume of information. The technologist will decide the plane to be viewed; for example, a stack of axial images reconstructed to demonstrate a sagittal image. In addition to displaying a different imaging plane, the technologist decides where the image plane is acquired; for example, a sagittal image 1 cm for the right lateral margin. The use of spiral imaging is the optimal method of acquiring a volume of information. This method ensures no gap in information for the reconstruction process.

The optimal MPR reconstruction is a result of optimal image acquisition before the reconstruction. The previous images should be contiguous with the same gantry tilt and the same field of view. Any alteration from this will result in degradation of the MPR image. It is important the images be attained free of motion artifact. MPR is a reconstruction process that uses image data. Therefore, MPR can be completed at a later time as long as the image data has been saved to an archiving device. The image detail of an MPR image is less than a conventional axial image. In addition, the reconstruction

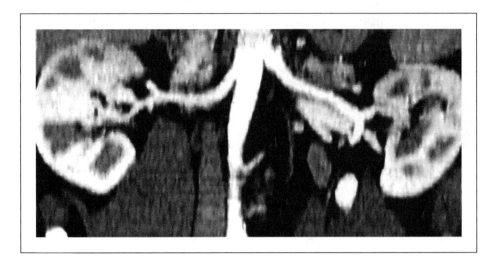

FIGURE 11-4

Image of multiplanar reconstruction of the kidneys.

process of a thin plane will result in better image detail when compared with a thick reconstruction plane (Fig. 11-4).

CT SPECIAL PROCEDURES FOR 3D VASCULAR RECONSTRUCTION (POSTPROCESSING ONLY)

Elective minimum required is 5.

Common Indications

- Presurgical evaluation of vascular structures and anomalies before resection
- Assessment of stenotic area within a vascular structure

Imaging Considerations

Three-dimensional imaging is the process of gathering a volume of information that is reconstructed into a model of information that can be rotated and surface rendered for visualization. The 3D image is a result of information gathered from the surface of anatomic structures. The technologist determines the surface to be reconstructed. This surface can range from the density of bone to the surface of vascular structures. The quality of the 3D reconstruction is highly dependent on the manner that the information previously was gathered. This information must be contiguous to produce a smooth 3D image without the stair-step appearance caused by disruption or lack of image information. The information is typically collected in one scan range at the same gantry angle and field of view throughout the entirety of the range. Spiral imaging is the ideal method of acquiring information for 3D reconstruction. CT angiography (CTA) uses the injection of contrast medium and the reconstruction of information into a 3D angiogram likeness. Because the contrast medium is injected intravenously, there is a reduction in reactions compared with the arterial bolus injection used in conventional angiography.

Before performing CTA, the technologist must have a firm understanding of the injection rate, injection duration, and delay after the injection to acquire the images at the optimal time. The optimal time to acquire the information is when the bolus of contrast medium passes through the region of interest. Because the circulation time of each patient can vary, a test ejection to determine ideal enhancement should be considered. This process involves a preliminary scan through the region of interest. The technologist positions the patient at the area of interest and a small sample of contrast medium (10–20 mL) is injected intravenously. This sample is injected at the same rate as the normal injection. After an 8-s delay, the technologist will scan serial images to determine the time of peak enhancement. This will then determine the accurate delay time for the individual's condition. Delay times range from 12 to 28 s for abdominal aorta and 10 to 20 s for the thoracic aorta.

The 3D image is formed by constructing an image from previously acquired information. The process takes the 2D information and views it from the desired direction. Typical viewing directions include frontal, lateral, posterior, superior, and inferior views. Current technology now allows the technologist to view the image at any increment or variation from the true anatomic position. The reconstruction process has several methods of using the acquired information. The method and use is determined by the software package available with each CT scanner and the methods acceptable to the physician's preference. At this time, the three methods of 3D reconstruction for vascular imaging include maximum intensity projection (MIP), shaded surface display (SSD), and curved plane reformatting (CPR). For the purpose of this manual, a general explanation of each method will be given. With each method, there are advantages and disadvantages. For this reason, the method or methods of choice are left to the imaging facility and the capabilities of the individual CT scanner.

In a general sense, the information on a 3D image should only include the area of interest. The goal is to display an image with the ideal spatial and contrast resolution. The use of a larger slice thickness and higher pitch during the spiral acquisition may be necessary to acquire all the information in the region of interest. A larger slice thickness and pitch will enable the entire region of interest to be acquired during a single breath hold of the patient. This method reduces volume imaging and slice misregistration caused by motion. To preserve the spatial resolution, the technologist should use a small field of view, which includes only the region of interest. However, many scanners will only allow for a reconstruction in the longitudinal plane equal to the distance of the FOV. Therefore, at times, the importance of the entire length of anatomy may require the technologist to select a larger FOV.

Reconstruction methods include the use of cropping tools for 3D images. Cropping tools will enable the technologist to exclude the undesired anatomy within or outside the region of interest. Cropping methods include physically tracing the area to be altered on the acquired axial images before the 3D reconstruction. There are two methods for cropping alterations. The first method will eliminate all information outside the traced area. The alternate method will eliminate the information within the traced area. Either method can eliminate problems such as overlapping information in areas such as the abdominal aorta superimposed over the spine. The advantages of each method include only reconstruction of the area of interest and visualization of only the area of interest. Both will reduce reconstruction times and unnecessary display of false or invalid information.

MAXIMUM INTENSITY PROJECTION (MIP)

The 3D image is a reconstructed creation as viewed from a specific plane, similar to when a person looks at the image from anterior to posterior plane. The image is created by a software manipulation that uses the maximal intensity value as if the image is projected to an image in the background of the view. This information is placed in the pixel location that corresponds to the view. This process is repeated until each pixel has the corresponding value associated with the view. The maximal intensity value is determined by setting the threshold at the desired value. This value in vascular imaging is equal to that of the bolus phase of contrast medium. This process displays the threshold value as white and everything below the value as dark. After the injection of contrast medium, the density of bone will be brighter than contrast medium. To accommodate this problem, the information from the bone processes can be eliminated by cropping or eliminating the underlying bone information. The software portion of the 3D reconstruction will allow the technologist to apply a border surrounding the area of interest. In this way, the data collected from the area of interest are the only information used to reconstruct the 3D image. This cropping method of elimination of unwanted information is actually a preprocessing step often used in CTA. In addition to eliminating the unwanted information, the reconstruction process is reduced because there is less information to work with.

Some negative results of MIP include the setting of the proper threshold. If the threshold is set to high, information from vascularity may be excluded in the images that were acquired before or after the bolus stage of contrast injection. Therefore, the accuracy of MIP is dependent on the threshold setting and ability to acquire the images at peak bolus stage of enhancement. Another hazard of MIP is the display of stenotic vessels. In smaller vessels with stenosis, the amount of contrast medium within the area is reduced. Because MIP uses the maximal intensity value, the areas of reduced flow will not be accurately displayed or will be lost due to partial volume effects. A final artifact of MIP is generated when the vessel orientation is oblique to the reconstructed image plane. When this event occurs, the information within the vessel will not be of maximum intensity. This will be displayed as a dotted line of information within the distal portion of the vessel. Because the size of vessel will increase the amount of intensity of the information, this artifact will be most notable in the distal end of small vessels.

SHADED SURFACE DISPLAY (SSD)

The SSD technique is an alternative to the MIP for developing an angiogram likeness. The SSD image displays the surface of the vessels. The appearance is similar to reflecting light off the object from the viewing direction. SSD involves the selection of a proper threshold value. Similar to MIP, the values above the threshold value will be displayed with the SSD manipulation. The selection of the proper threshold will also influence the image reconstruction. The proper threshold should be set to include the shades of gray that will include areas that are slightly outside the bolus phase. Improper high threshold settings can reduce the appearance of stenotic or the distal ends of smaller vessels. A low threshold setting can increase the amount of noise, and higher density soft tissue will obscure the desired vasculature.

CURVED PLANE REFORMATTING (CPR)

The principle behind CPR is to extract information from the surface of the area of interest. The technologist can trace around the area of interest that previously has been acquired through MIP. The CPR software program then extracts the information within the traced area and interpolates the remaining pixels. CPR produces an image that is only one pixel thick instead of an image created from multiple layers of pixel values. CPR is very operator dependent and is subject to loss of information caused by improper tracing that can eliminate too much information. In addition, because the remaining pixel values must be used for the resulting image, there is a large amount of interpolation completed between the remaining pixels. This process will result in a reduction of spatial resolution.

The technologist must be aware of the pitfalls that accompany the choice of 3D reconstruction methods or submethods. For the ideal 3D vascular image, the use of the smallest field of view that includes only the area of interest will improve the resulting spatial resolution. The use of a soft or standard algorithm will improve the contrast resolution. Trying to scan only the length of the area of interest that simultaneously can be completed in a single breath hold will normally allow for the optimal reconstruction into a 3D image. The technologist must remember that the goal is to acquire an image that resembles an angiogram. The CT process to accomplish this is very dependent on the pre-examination preparations and the choice of reconstruction.

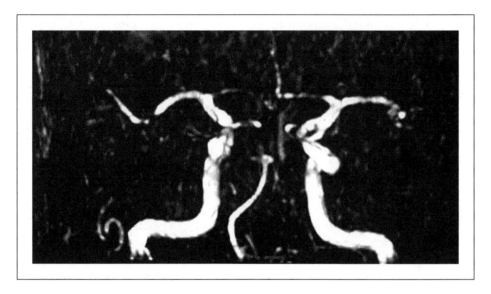

FIGURE 11-5

Image of 3D vascular reconstruction of the circle of Willis.

The radiologist's preference and department standard will have the largest influence on the method of reconstruction. In summary, the presence of motion will distract from the image quality before any reconstruction efforts. The technologist can only reconstruct a 3D image of quality equal to the quality of the information available before the reconstruction (Fig. 11-5).

CT SPECIAL PROCEDURES FOR 3D BONE RECONSTRUCTION (POSTPROCESSING ONLY)

Elective minimum required is 5.

Common Indications

- Presurgical evaluation of bony structures and anomalies
- Evaluation for uses in craniofacial surgery and orthopedics
- Planning for radiation therapy

Imaging Considerations

3D imaging is the process of gathering a volume of information that is reconstructed into a model of information that can be rotated and surface rendered for visualization. The 3D image is a result of information gathered from the surface of anatomic structures. The technologist will determine the surface to be reconstructed. This surface can range from the density of bone to the surface of vascular structures. The quality of the 3D reconstruction is highly dependent on the manner that the information previously was gathered. This information must be contiguous to produce a smooth 3D image without the stair-step appearance caused by disruption or lack of image information. The information is typically collected in one scan range at the same gantry angle and same field of view throughout the entirety of the range. Spiral imaging is the ideal method of acquiring information for 3D reconstruction.

The 3D image is formed by constructing the image from previously acquired information. The process takes the 2D information and views it from a desired direction. The reconstruction process has several methods of using the acquired information. The method and use is determined by the software package available with each CT scanner and the methods acceptable to the physician's preference. At this time, the three methods of 3D reconstruction for bony imaging include MIP, SSD, and CPR. For the purpose of this manual, a general explanation of each method will be given. With each method there are advantages and disadvantages; for this reason, the method or methods of choice are left to the imaging facility and the capabilities of the individual CT scanner.

In a general sense, the information of a 3D image should only include the area of interest. The goal is to display an image with the ideal spatial and contrast resolution. The use of a larger slice thickness and higher pitch during the spiral acquisition may be necessary to acquire all the information through the region of interest. A larger slice thickness and pitch will enable the entire region of interest to be acquired during a single breath hold of the patient. This method reduces volume imaging and slice misregistration caused by motion. To preserve the spatial resolution, the technologist should use a small field of view, which includes only the region of interest. Many scanners will only allow for a reconstruction in the longitudinal plane equal to the distance of the FOV. Therefore, at times the importance of the entire length of anatomy may require the technologist to select a larger FOV.

Reconstruction methods include the use of cropping tools for 3D images. Cropping tools will enable the technologist to exclude the undesired anatomy within or outside the region of interest. Cropping methods include physically tracing the area to alter on the acquired axial images. There are two methods for cropping alterations. The first method will eliminate everything outside the traced area. The alternate method will eliminate the information within the traced area. Either method can eliminate problems such as overlapping information in areas such as the abdominal aorta superimposed over the spine. The advantages of each method include reconstruction of the area of interest and visualization of only the area of interest. Both methods will reduce reconstruction times and unnecessary display of false or invalid information.

MAXIMUM INTENSITY PROJECTION

The 3D image is a reconstructed creation as viewed from a specific plane, similar to when a person looks at the image from anterior to posterior plane. The image is created by a software manipulation that uses the maximal intensity Hounsfield value as if the image were projected to an image in the background of the view. This information is placed in the pixel location that corresponds to the view. The process is repeated until each pixel has the corresponding value associated with the view. The maximal intensity value is determined by setting the threshold at the desired value. This value in bony imaging is set at approximately +150 Hounsfield units. This process displays the threshold value as white and everything below the value as dark. Three-dimensional reconstruction is often more successful at discriminating bony surfaces and skin surfaces than at distinguishing the layers of muscle and fascial layers, because the difference in Hounsfield units is greater between skin and air or between soft tissue and bone in typical scanning.

Some of the negative results of MIP include the setting of the proper threshold. If the threshold is set to low, information from unwanted soft tissue may be included in the resulting image.

SHADED SURFACE DISPLAY

The SSD technique is an alternative to the MIP for developing an anatomic likeness. The SSD image displays the surface of the vessels. The appearance is similar to reflecting light off the object from the viewing direction. SSD also involves the selection of a proper threshold value. Similar to MIP, the values above the threshold value will be displayed with the SSD manipulation. The selection of the proper threshold will also influence the image reconstruction. Similar pitfalls accompany improper threshold values of SSD as with MIP imaging.

CURVED PLANE REFORMATTING

The principle behind CPR is to extract information from the surface of the area of interest. The technologist can trace around the area of interest that previously has been acquired through MIP. The CPR software program then extracts the information within the traced area and interpolates the remaining pixels. CPR produces an image that is only one pixel thick instead of an image created from multiple layers of pixel values. CPR is very operator dependent and is subject to loss of information caused by improper tracing that can eliminate too much information. Because the remaining pixel values must be used for the resulting image, there is a large amount of interpolation completed between the remaining pixels. This process will result in a reduction of spatial resolution.

The technologist must be aware of the pitfalls that accompany the choice of 3D reconstruction method or submethod. For the ideal 3D

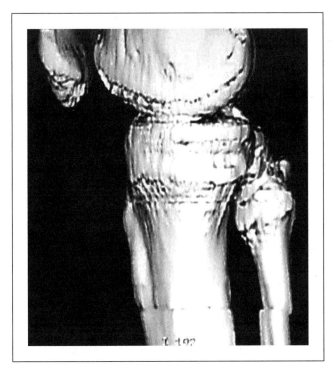

FIGURE 11-6

Image of 3D bone reconstruction of the knee.

bony image, the use of the smallest field of view that will still include the area of interest will improve the resulting spatial resolution. The use of a soft or standard algorithm will improve the contrast resolution. Trying to scan only the length of the area of interest that simultaneously can be completed in a single breath hold will normally allow for the optimal reconstruction into a 3D image. The technologist must remember that the goal is to acquire an image that resembles a true anatomic structure. The CT process to accomplish this is very dependent on the pre-examination preparations and the choice of reconstruction. The radiologist's preference and department standard will have the largest influence on the method of reconstruction. In summary, the presence of motion will distract from the image quality before any reconstruction efforts. The technologist can only reconstruct a 3D image of quality equal to the quality of the information available before the reconstruction (Fig. 11-6).

CT SPECIAL PROCEDURES FOR 3D VIRTUAL REALITY (FLY THROUGH, NAVIGATOR; INCLUDING POSTPROCESSING)

Elective minimum required is 3. This protocol must be completed on a patient, not a simulation.

Common Indications

- Endoluminal evaluation for surgical planning
- Realistic animations
- Virtual laparoscopy
- Virtual endoscopy

Imaging Considerations

Three-dimensional virtual reality is a software program designed for the reconstruction of information to display interluminal structures. This method of reconstruction will allow for an endoscopic appearance of structures such as colon, trachea, bronchi, urinary tract, or any potential lesion within the lumen. The software program uses a surface or volume rendering process that allows for the visualization of the lumen surface only. The resulting image is similar to cutting a section out of a pipe and visualizing the inside of the pipe surface from within the lumen. In addition, the software program allows the technologist to follow the course of the lumen, allowing for the complete inspection for the distance of the reconstruction. The images are reconstructed from previously acquired images and displayed in a real-time format. Spiral images attained provide optimal information for the reconstruction of virtual images. Virtual software allows the technologist to alter the surface appearance with color and shades to enhance the appearance and simulate a conventional endoscopic appearance.

The basic concept of virtual reality is to eliminate the undesired information within the lumen of interest. The challenge is to identify the threshold values that will eliminate the information such as air and still leave the desired information of the lumen wall. This process is completed by surface rendering or volume rendering. Because the view is similar to being within the lumen, the pixels located closest to the viewer will have a blocky appearance and the pixels viewed as a distance for the view will have a normal high-resolution appearance. With continual improvement in spatial resolution in conventional CT scanning, the spatial resolution of 3D virtual imaging will also improve.

Virtual reality provides an alternative to the conventional methods of colonoscopy, endoscopy, and bronchoscopy. Three-dimensional virtual imaging allows for accurate geometric and densitometric information concerning the areas within the lumen. Software is now available to allow the technologist to view the lumen wall as transparent. This option allows the technologist to evaluate the structures adjacent to the lumen. The virtual process is less invasive and traumatic to the patient than the conventional bronchoscopy procedure. There are no medical complications involved with virtual bronchoscopy, because it is a postprocessing reconstruction program.

Virtual reality programs still allow the physician to view segments of the lumen with the appearance similar to those from a bronchoscopy or endoscopy procedure. Three-dimensional virtual reality now provides the information to evaluate the structure before surgery, without further traumatizing the patient.

NONIMAGING AND QUALITY ASSURANCE PROCEDURES IN CT

CHAPTER 12

CT Experience and Patient Care

	Mandatory
Patient care	
Vital signs	5
CPR	Certification
Universal precautions	5
O_2 administration	3
Assessment and monitoring level of consciousness and respiration	5
Assessment for contraindication for procedure	5
Sterile technique	3
Verify informed consent when necessary	3

CT EXPERIENCE REQUIREMENTS CONCERNING PROCEDURES REQUIRING THE KNOWLEDGE OF VITAL SIGNS (BLOOD PRESSURE, PULSE, RESPIRATION, TEMPERATURE)

Mandatory minimum required is 5.

Common Indications

- A change in the patient's condition
- Taken before and after any interventional or invasive diagnostic procedure

Imaging Considerations

Vital signs consist of measurement and monitoring of the patient's current blood pressure, pulse, respiration, and temperature values. These rates are compared with the rate or value of the average person in the same age category or preferable to the patient's previous values. The technologist should be aware of the normal values for each of the vital signs and be proficient in the assessment of the values. The vital signs are normally taken as a series but will be discussed on an individual basis.

BLOOD PRESSURE

Blood pressure readings are created by the arterial pressure against the vessel wall. This is equivalent to the amount of pressure to push mercury in a sphygmomanometer one millimeter. This force is a result of the contractive phase of the left ventricle pushing blood into the aorta. At peak compression the heart will have the maximum force. This is termed the systolic phase of the heart. During the process of relaxation of the ventricle, the pressure will drop to the minimal force; this is the diastolic phase. The blood pressure value is normally charted as systolic over diastolic values. The average blood pressure value is 120/80 mmHg. Hypertension occurs when a patient's systolic value is above 140 and/or the diastolic value is above 90 mmHg. Hypotension occurs when the systolic pressure is below 90 mmHg and only 10 mmHg in the diastolic phase.

Blood pressures are taken with the use of an aneroid or mercury manometer and a stethoscope. The aneroid manometer (blood pressure cuff) comes in a variety of sizes. The appropriate cuff should fit the patient and body part. The technologist should always wash his or her hands before taking the patient's blood pressure. The patient should be positioned with the arm extended. Normally, the blood pressure is taken with the cuff wrapped around the patient's arm, approximately 1 in. superior to the antecubital space. This places the cuff over the area of the brachial artery. The cuff should be wrapped snugly around the patient's arm, with the air valve open and the cuff deflated. The air valve should now be closed and the cuff inflated. As the cuff is inflated, the technologist should be able to palpate the brachial or radial artery. Inflation of the cuff should continue until the meter reads 30 mmHg above the point where the pulse disappears. The cuff should be slowly deflated by releasing the air valve; the technologist should note the point where the pulse becomes apparent. Continue to deflate the cuff and wait approximately thirty seconds to allow venous flow to prevent a false reading. This time the process is repeated with the diaphragm of the stethoscope placed over the brachial artery. Close the air valve and reinflate the cuff to the level where 30 mmHg is above the systolic point. Slowly release the valve allowing the mercury to fall at a rate of 2 to 3 mmHg/s. The systolic level is the point where the first clear pulsation sound appears. Continue releasing the cuff at the same rate until the pulsation sound disappears; this is the diastolic reading. Upon completion of the blood pressure readings, completely deflate and remove the cuff. The technologist should wash his or her hands before entering the blood pressure levels. Record the levels in the proper space on the chart and evaluate the readings compared with previous levels and department standards.

PULSE

A pulse is present every time the left ventricle is contracted and forces blood into the arterial system. We can feel the presence of the pulse when we compress an artery against underlying muscle or bone structures. Pulse is frequently monitored on the medial side of the wrist in the area of the radial artery. When the body experiences a life-threatening situation, the body senses the need for the blood flow to the brain. This event may make the location of the pulse in the radial artery difficult. Other locations to monitor the pulse are the areas of the brachial, axilla, and carotid arteries. The peripheral blood circulation will usually decrease with an increase in life-threatening situations.

The technologist should wash his or her hands before taking the pulse of a patient. At the radial artery location, the technologist should place his or her thumb on the posterior side of the patient's wrist area. This method allows the technologist to place his or her fingers on the anterior side of the patient's wrist over the radial artery. Lightly put pressure on the radial artery until the pulse is felt. Count the pulses for 15 s and then multiply the number of pulses by 4. This product is the pulse rate occurring in 1 min. The pulse rate should be charted and compared with the patient's normal rate or department standards. In addition, the pulse rate should be reported as normal, slow, rapid, weak, or irregular.

RESPIRATION

Respiration is the normal exchange process occurring between the alveoli and red blood cells within the lungs. A visible full respiration cycle is from the point the patient has one complete inspiration and one complete expiration. When assessing the respiration of a patient, the technologist is assessing the breathing rate, depth, and rhythm. The process is charted as the number of cycles occurring in 1 min, if the process involved shallow or normal breaths that were consistent or variable and if the respiration process was labored or not. Under normal conditions, it takes little conscious effort on the patient's part to complete the respiration process. When the patient has a noticeable effort in breathing, the technologist can visibly observe a pronounced movement of the neck, shoulders, and chest muscles. Checking respiration rate is normally a visual test, in which the technologist inconspicuously observes the person breathing. This monitoring continues for 15 s, and the number of cycles is then multiplied by 4 to attain the number of cycles per min. Checking respiration can be completed when checking the patient's pulse rate. The technologist should always be alert when there is a sudden change in a patient's respiration. Respiratory distress may occur when patients have a sudden change in respiration rate, depth, or rhythm. In this event, the technologist should notify the physician.

TEMPERATURE

The normal temperature of the human body is 37°C (98.6°F). Exercise, disease, infection, or exposure to extreme warm or cold conditions can make temperatures occur above or below the normal value. Temperatures in the diagnostic imaging department are normally checked orally. If the patient is at risk or unable to place a thermometer in the mouth, the option of an axillary measurement or tympanic-membrane measurement is possible. Current electronic thermometers are convenient and safe for oral and axillary monitoring of temperature. The technologist should be aware of the proper oral or axillary use. Tympanic membrane measurements are convenient for pediatric patients. The technologist should be aware of the proper use of all thermometers kept within the facility.

CT EXPERIENCE DEMONSTRATING THE PROPER USE OF UNIVERSAL PRECAUTIONS

Mandatory requirements of 5 procedures.

Common Indications

- Precautionary actions to avoid the accidental spread of HIV, hepatitis B, or both
- Protect the health care worker from bloodborne pathogens

Universal Precautions

Universal precautions provide the health care worker with a consistent set of guidelines to avoid contamination from bloodborne pathogens. The Occupational Safety and Health Administration defines universal precautions as the minimal standard for safety with concern to bloodborne pathogens. The recommendation of the U.S. Department of Health and Human Services for universal precautions is to treat every patient as a potential carrier of HIV or hepatitis B infection.

It is common practice to use universal precautions consistently for every patient the technologist is in contact with. To ensure the continual practice of universal precautions, the health care worker is periodically reoriented and evaluated on the standards. Each imaging facility should have a complete list of universal precautions to use as a reference before examination of patients. The following is a list of standard universal practices with which the technologist should be proficient.

- The use of gloves is probably the easiest and most frequently used precaution in imaging departments. Gloves should be worn whenever there is potential for contact with infectious organisms from bodily fluids. The technologist should routinely use gloves when in contact with blood, bodily fluids, or nonintact skin. The potential for needle sticks is another precaution involving the contamination of blood or other bodily fluids. The use of latex gloves has proven slightly more protective when compared with vinyl gloves in the prevention of puncture from needle sticks. Gloves should be changed after contact with each patient. Upon completion of the examination or saturation of the gloves, the technologist should remove the gloves and dispose of them in the proper container to avoid future contact with other health care workers. After disposal of gloves, the health care worker should use appropriate handwashing techniques.

- Masks and protective facewear should be used when the potential for contact of any bloodborne pathogen exists. Certain procedures require the placement of catheters and the frequent risk of contact with bodily fluids. During every invasive situation, the technologist should wear protective eyewear that guards from frontal and side exposure to the eyes.

- The use of gowns and protective eyewear may be necessary to complete a procedure that may involve blood or bodily fluids. Protective gowns should be long enough to cover all of your clothing, should be long sleeved, and have tight-fitting cuffs. Impermeable gowns or aprons must be worn during any procedure with potential of contamination from blood or other bodily fluids. Gowns should be removed after saturation or completion of examination. Gowns should be placed in the proper disposal container to avoid contact with other health care workers.

- The technologist should *not* attempt to recap needles at the completion of use. Needles should not be removed from the syringe for purposes of disposal of the needle. Needles should be properly disposed of upon completion of use. Puncture-proof biohazard containers designed for the disposal of needles, should not be overfilled or left with needles protruding the open container. After the completion of the examination, the technologist should properly wash his or her hands.

- The technologist should immediately wash his or her hands or other skin surfaces after the contamination of blood or other bodily fluids. The use of proper washing techniques should be used.

- The use of ventilation devices, mouthpieces, and Ambu bags should be used instead of direct mouth-to-mouth resuscitation.

- Health care providers with open or oozing sores should abstain from direct contact and handling of patients or equipment.

CT EXPERIENCE DEMONSTRATING THE PROPER ADMINISTRATION OF OXYGEN

Mandatory requirements of 3 procedures.

Common Indications

- Prevent or minimize the increased cardiopulmonary workload
- Correct hypoxemia or suspected tissue hypoxia

Imaging Considerations

Hypoxemia is an insufficient oxygenation of the blood supply. Hypoxia is the deficiency of oxygen or a decrease in the oxygen content in inspired air. The tissues most sensitive to hypoxia are the brain, heart, lungs, and liver. To compensate for hypoxia, the blood pressure, respiratory depth, and respiratory rate will increase. A hypoxic patient may struggle during respiration and exhibit a shortness of breath. For these reasons, patients arriving for the CT examination may require the additional use of oxygen. Oxygen is considered a medication, and like any medication, oxygen does have positive and negative affects. Because oxygen is considered a medication, a physician must prescribe it to patients. The technologist may be required to assist in the changing or the administration of oxygen for the patient in the computed tomography department. It is the responsibility of the technologist to be aware of the location of portable supplies and permanent locations for the administration of oxygen. The administration of oxygen is a normal process for the respiratory department of the facility, but it is also the responsibility of the technologist to be competent in the administration of oxygen while the patient is in the imaging department.

Oxygen administration is measured in liters of oxygen per minute (L O_2/min). Oxygen mixes with room air when administered; therefore, the percentage of oxygen can vary with respiratory rate and efficiency of the patient. Oxygen supplies typically are permanent as from a wall outlet and flow meter or portable from an oxygen cylinder and regulator. The supply of oxygen to wall outlets originates within the facility and is piped throughout the necessary departments and patient rooms. Administration of oxygen involves alternate methods of mixing room air and oxygen. The amounts and type of oxygen administration is dependent on the patient needs and type of delivery device prescribed by the physician. The oxygen administration used within the radiology department uses low to moderate concentrations of oxygen. Patients with a mechanical ventilator who are in need of a CT procedure should be accompanied by someone from the respiratory department to monitor the patient's condition.

Oxygen may be administered through either a nasal cannula or oxygen mask. The nasal cannula administers oxygen through a plastic tubing device placed so the outlet ports are within the nasal entrance. Nasal cannulas are used to administer 24 to 36% oxygen at a rate 1 to 4 L O_2/min. The use of a nasal cannula for long periods has the tendency to dry the patient's nasal mucous membranes and cause nasal congestion. Fluid moisturizers may be attached at the oxygen source to reduce this problem.

Simple oxygen masks fit over the patient's mouth and nose. Simple oxygen masks are designed for a mixture of room air and oxygen. The patient can expel the air back into the mask and through vents into the room with this type of mask. The use of a simple oxygen mask is for short periods of time. The efficiency of the oxygen administration mask is dependent on the seal surrounding the mask. This type of mask is used to administer 35% to 60% oxygen at a rate of 4 to 6 L O_2/min.

Nonrebreather masks are for delivering high concentrations of oxygen. A single directional valve will not allow the expired air to mix with the incoming air supply. Vents are located on the sides of the nonrebreather mask to allow the expired air to pass outside of the mask. There is a plastic reservoir bag attached to the nonrebreather mask. The supply of oxygen is contained within the reservoir. When the patient expels the air, the valve closes on the reservoir and prevents the mixture of carbon dioxide with the incoming oxygen. When the patient inhales, the valve on the reservoir bag opens and allows the volume of oxygen to flow. The masks should maintain a volume flow that will allow for the reservoir to remain filled. Nonrebreather masks can deliver a mixture of between 55% and 90% oxygen.

Patients with chronic obstructive pulmonary disease may require the use of a Venturi mask. These masks are designed for the patient who cannot tolerate high oxygen concentrations. The velocity of the oxygen is increased by forcing it through a small opening in the mask. The mask pulls room air into the mask to mix with the incoming oxygen. A Venturi mask will allow the percentage of oxygen to be set at specific levels from 24% to 50%.

When the patient arrives at the imaging department with oxygen treatment present, the technologist must not remove the oxygen supply unless authorized by the physician. The technologist must exercise care to avoid tangling or pulling on oxygen supply tubing when transporting the patient from wheel chairs and cart to the examination table. The technologist must also be aware of the locations of oxygen supplies and methods of oxygen treatment. An oxygen valve from wall or temporary sources should not be left open when not in use, because oxygen supports combustion. In addition portable oxygen cylinders are pressurized to 2000 lb/in^2. The technologist, therefore, must avoid tipping or dropping cylinders. Damage to regulators or cylinders may occur from dropping or abusive contact.

CT EXPERIENCE DEMONSTRATING PATIENT ASSESSMENT AND MONITORING LEVEL OF CONSCIOUSNESS AND RESPIRATION

Mandatory requirements of 5 procedures.

Common Indications

- Assessment for sudden changes in a patient's neurologic function

Imaging Considerations

Most patients will not require special monitoring during the CT examination. Inpatients which are scheduled for a CT examination normally have a baseline of vital signs charted. Outpatients arriving to the computed tomography department typically do not have the baseline of vital signs. During the initial assessment of the patient's condition, it may be necessary for the technologist to collect the vital signs to serve for future comparison in the event that changes occur in the patient's mental or neurologic status. During the initial assessment, the technologist should notice the patient's condition regarding anxiety, speech, personality, and respiration. A patient can initially have normal breathing and change to shallow or labored respiration. For example, a patient with head injuries can go from a normal state and deteriorate to a slow pulse and respiratory rate. If the patient's condition changes, the technologist may need to stop the examination and summon immediate assistance from a physician.

The technologist should monitor for different levels of consciousness. Levels of consciousness can range from completely alert to nonresponsive. The patient may seem irritable and uncooperative as they change levels of consciousness. The technologist should note any response changes as they occur. A patient is considered conscious and alert if he or she can respond to questions and other stimuli. Patients who display a drowsy appearance but may still be aroused through loud speech or gentle physical contact are considered more serious than the alert patient. The most serious condition exists when the technologist cannot arouse the patient through verbal attempts or physical stimuli.

The level of consciousness can be assessed by asking the patient for information and by his or her ability to follow verbal instructions. The technologist should ask the patient to state his or her name, the date, his or her address, and the reason he or she has come to the imaging department. If the responses are correct and completed in an adequate amount of time, it should be noted that the patient responds to verbal stimuli. The technologist should note any delay in responses or need for repetition of questions. If the patient responds in an irritable manner or struggles with the proper choice of words, the technologist should note the patient's condition. When instructing the patient on the positioning for the examination, note the patient's ability to follow the instructions. When the patient is moving, the technologist should note any movement or position that causes pain or deviation from attention. These observations will create a baseline for comparison in the patient's neurologic and mental status for later assessment.

The Glasgow Coma Scale is a method for the rapid assessment of neurologic function and level of response. The areas of evaluation include eye opening, motor response, and verbal response. The Glasgow Scale assigns a numerical value to evaluate the patient's neurologic status in each area. The higher the overall score on the scale, the higher the level of conscious functioning. The highest possible score of the Glasgow Coma Scale is 15 (Table 12-1).

TABLE 12-1

Glasgow Coma Scale

Action	Response	Score
Eyes open		
	Spontaneously	4
	To speech	3
	To pain	2
	None	1
Best verbal response		
	Oriented	5
	Confused	4
	Inappropriate words	3
	Incomprehensible sounds	2
	None	1
Best motor response		
	Obeys commands	6
	Localized pain	5
	Flexion withdrawal	4
	Abnormal flexion	3
	Abnormal extension	2
	Flaccid	1
Highest possible score		15

CT EXPERIENCE DEMONSTRATING PATIENT ASSESSMENT FOR CONTRAINDICATIONS OF A CT EXAMINATION

Mandatory requirements of 5 procedures.

Common Indications

- Assessment for conditions that may alter the normal CT procedure or cause reason for an alternative examination by another imaging modality

Imaging Considerations

The beginning of each CT examination should start with the assessment of whether the CT examination is the appropriate examination for the patient's specific needs. According to Taber's cyclopedic medical dictionary, a contraindication is any symptom or circumstance indicating the inappropriateness of a form of treatment otherwise advisable. Reasons for contraindications of a CT examination include pregnancy, allergic reactions to contrast medium used in computed tomography, and laboratory values outside the acceptable levels for intravenous contrast injections or interventional procedures. The above-mentioned list may be a permanent or a temporary contraindication for a CT examination. A contraindication for a CT examination is based largely on past experiences of the radiologist, imaging facility, and recommendations by the contrast manufacturer.

The appropriate patient history concerning the CT examination should include questions of pregnancy, previous surgeries, allergies, and history of asthma. The technologist should attain current information involving laboratory values for patients scheduled for interventional procedures and any other procedure requiring the use of contrast medium. For the purpose of this book, each contraindication will be discussed in a general sense. The technologist should investigate specific areas within the book (e.g., assessment of vital signs, evaluation of lab values, and contrast agent selection) concerning proper methods of use and contraindications.

CONTRAINDICATIONS OF A CT EXAMINATION INVOLVING PREGNANT PATIENTS

CT examinations during the first trimester of a pregnancy should be rescheduled for a later date if possible. Exposure to radiation during the first trimester of pregnancy is associated with a dramatic increase in prenatal death and abnormalities compared with radiation exposure during the second and third trimester. An ultrasound examination during the first trimester may be one alternative to computed tomography. The benefits from the CT examination should always be compared with the risk involved, especially in cases of pregnancy. Some imaging facilities may require patients of childbearing years to wait for the CT examination until the next menstrual period unless they are certain they are not pregnant. Each imaging facility will have its own specific protocol involving the CT examination of pregnant patients. The technologist should be aware of the specific protocol and any additional shielding required for the examination.

CONTRAINDICATIONS OF A CT EXAMINATION INVOLVING CONTRAST MEDIUM

Contrast medium is frequently used as part of the CT examination. Contrast medium can be ingested, injected, or introduced rectally. If the patient is allergic to any type of contrast medium, it is necessary to understand alternatives and possible premedication methods available. Some physicians will not approve of certain CT examinations without the use of contrast medium. For example, oral contrast medium is used for opacification of bowel. The lack of bowel opacification jeopardizes the value of the gathered information. A diluted version of barium sulfate is the common choice of bowel opacification. However if the patient is allergic to barium or suspected of gastrointestinal perforation, the use of barium sulfate solution is contraindicated. The alternative would be to use a water soluble iodinated contrast medium or possibly to have an MRI, or ultrasound examination.

Many CT examinations require the use of iodinated intravenous contrast medium. If the patient is allergic to the contrast medium, it may be possible to treat the allergy with a premedication regime starting 48 h before the examination. This alternative is specific to the imaging facility. Another alternative is to schedule an ultrasound or MRI instead of the CT examination.

CONTRAINDICATIONS OF A CT EXAMINATION INVOLVING LABORATORY VALUES

Patients with elevated blood urea and nitrogen (BUN) level, creatine level, or both, may need to postpone or reschedule the portion of the examination requiring the use of injectable contrast medium. Patients may need to be rescheduled for a CT-assisted aspiration, drainage, or biopsy procedure if the platelet count, prothrombin time (PT), or partial thromboplastin time (PTT) levels are not within the acceptable limits. Patients can typically reschedule the CT examination once the laboratory values are within the acceptable limits.

CONTRAINDICATIONS OF A CT EXAMINATION INVOLVING THE PATIENT'S VITAL SIGNS

The normal CT examination does not require the assistance of other individuals outside the radiology department. In the case of a patient whose vital signs are outside the acceptable limits, the use of ancillary assistance may be necessary. At times, personnel from the respiratory and nursing departments may be necessary for successful completion of the CT examination. With the additional support personnel involved, it is the technologist's responsibility to ensure proper radiation precautions are followed. In cases for which stabilizing the patient's condition is not possible, the CT examination may need to be canceled or rescheduled.

CT EXPERIENCE DEMONSTRATING STERILE TECHNIQUES

Mandatory requirements of 3 procedures.

Common Indications

- Providing direct assistance to the radiologist and support personnel during a sterile procedure in conjunction with a CT examination

Imaging Considerations

The technologist will typically operate the CT scanner throughout the imaging procedure. At times the technologist may be required to directly assist the radiologist during an interventional procedure; therefore, the technologist must be equally proficient at sterile techniques as part of the qualification of operating the CT scanner. During any sterile procedure, the number of people directly involved in the procedure should be kept to a minimum. The patient, radiologist, technologist, and support personnel to directly assist the radiologist are the minimal number involved during a sterile procedure. If the radiologist has direct assistance, the assistant will don sterile apparel and directly assist in the sterile procedure. The direct assistant will be considered sterile, and the technologist operating the CT scanner will be considered the unsterile person. In this case, the technologist will be responsible for operating the CT scanner and assisting the radiologist and support person by providing necessary or additional items that may become necessary during the examination process.

The technologist should be aware of the specific requirements involving sterile techniques. Sterile techniques or surgical asepsis is the elimination of pathogens by sterilization. Medical and surgical asepsis is practiced in the computed tomography department during cases of interventional procedures such as biopsies, aspirations, and drainage. The technologist may need to directly assist the radiologist throughout the sterile procedure. In this case, the technologist must be proficient in each of the above categories. When the technologist does not directly assist the radiologist, the technologist will need to be proficient at assisting without fear of contamination of the sterile field or other support personnel. The CT technologist should have a thorough understanding of sterile technique involving the proper gowning and washing, preparation of the sterile field, and maintenance of the sterile field.

Once a sterile package is opened, only necessary personnel should be allowed in the room to avoid accidental contamination of the sterile field. Doors entering the procedure room should remain closed to avoid contamination by airborne pathogens. The sterile person assisting the radiologist should avoid turning away from the sterile field. The area below the waist of the sterile person is considered contaminated. The unsterile personnel should avoid leaning across or passing of any unsterile objects over the sterile field. The success of any sterile procedure is centered around the organization of the technologist and assisting personnel. The area within the examination room should remain uncluttered and organized. Organization will avoid accidental contamination of sterile persons or sterile field. Organization will also reduce unnecessary stress during the examination process.

Sterile packages should be used before the expiration date. If the package does not contain an expiration date, it should not be used. Any sterile package found to be torn open, wet, or damaged is considered unsterile. Sterile packages should be opened just before the procedure, to avoid accidental contamination. A sterile field is created once the package is opened. The outer 1-in. border of an opened sterile package is considered a contaminated area. Other sterile objects should be dropped on to the sterile field or placed on the field with the assistance of sterile forceps. When using liquids, the first part of the liquid should be poured into a waste receptacle to wash bacteria from the lip of the bottle. The remaining contents of the bottle should be poured into a sterile container without making contact between the bottle and sterile container. If an unsterile object makes contact with a sterile object, the sterile object will now be considered unsterile. Whenever there is a question regarding an object being contaminated, the technologist should consider it contaminated.

CT EXPERIENCE DEMONSTRATING VERIFICATION OF INFORMED CONSENT WHEN NECESSARY

Mandatory requirements of 3 procedures.

Common Indications

- Providing complete information about a specific examination, including risks, benefits, and alternatives to the examination
- Assurance that the information concerning the examination is understood before the examination is to begin.

Imaging Considerations

Informed consent is when a patient agrees to participate in an examination such as a biopsy or other interventional procedure. This agreement is based on the factual information about the examination. The factual information should include risks and benefits of the procedure. Patients should also be informed of any alternative methods to the procedure. In addition to informing the patient on the possible CT procedure, the technologist must be assured that the patient or representative of the patient understands the information completely. Only after all information concerning the examination is given and the assurance that the information is understood should the patient be asked to sign the consent form. The autonomy of the patient should always be of concern before performing any diagnostic examination.

Signed consent forms routinely are necessary before any invasive, interventional, or potentially hazardous procedure. If the patient is not of legal age or capable of understanding or signing the consent form, a legal representative is allowed to sign for the patient. In most cases, the physician is the responsible party for obtaining the consent.

General consent forms that a patient signs during admission to a care facility are not the same as a consent form for a diagnostic examination. Consent forms are often specific to the imaging facility and examination procedure. In the event that a consent form for the examination has been completed before the patient entered the radiology department, the technologist must be sure that the information is correct before the examination. Some informed consent forms will allow space for the patient to write the process of the examination in his or her own words. This method provides the physician with a certain amount of proof that the patient does understand the examination that they are about to undergo. Typical information on consent forms should include the following:

Name of the imaging facility

Date and time of explanation of examination

Name of referring physician

Type of CT procedure to be performed

Complications and benefits of the procedures

A clause allowing the physician surgical permission to alleviate an unforeseen complication

Name of the physician explaining the procedure

Signature of patient or legal representative

Signature of witness observing the explanation process

Some imaging facilities require the completion of a consent form before any CT examination requiring the use of contrast medium. It is the responsibility of the technologist to understand the specific department policy involving the use of consent forms.

CHAPTER 13

Performing Contrast Administration Procedures (i.e., Intravenous, Oral, Rectal, Catheter)

The procedure marked with an asterisk may be demonstrated by performing all steps excluding those involving actual skin puncture in states or institutions where venipuncture by registered technologists is prohibited.

Procedure	Mandatory
Evaluation of laboratory values before procedure	5
Contrast agent selection	5
Contrast agent preparation	5
Site selection	5
Venipuncture*	5
Power injector	5
Monitoring patient for adverse reaction	5

CT EXPERIENCE REQUIREMENTS FOR PROCEDURES REQUIRING THE EVALUATION OF LABORATORY VALUES BEFORE PROCEDURE (BUN, CREATININE)

Mandatory minimum required is 5.

Common Indications

- Assessment of available laboratory values before the use of contrast medium
- Assessment of the patient's renal function before the use of contrast medium
- Assessment of the patient's ability of the blood to coagulate before a CT-assisted interventional procedure

Imaging Considerations

Contrast medium is frequently used for the localization of a lesion. The CT examination of the abdomen and pelvis frequently will require the use of oral contrast medium be used for the opacification of bowel. Intravenous contrast medium is used in studies of the abdomen and pelvis to differentiate between adjacent vessels and to determine the vascularity of the lesion. Contrast medium can be directly injected into cysts to reveal the true dimensions of the structure. For these reasons, it is vital for the technologist to understand the laboratory tests and associated values before any CT procedure requiring the use of contrast medium.

An associated risk in a biopsy procedure is from bleeding. This risk is increased with the type and diameter of biopsy needle and with increased vascularity of the lesion. Patients with bleeding disorders may be contraindicated for a biopsy procedure, unless treatment for the disorder is completed before the biopsy. Because bleeding is a risk of any interventional procedure, the technologist should be familiar with laboratory tests evaluating the ability of the patient's blood to clot.

Before the examination, the technologist must be aware of the department standards concerning the laboratory values and signed consent forms associated with the use of contrast medium. Before the use of intravenous contrast medium, the technologist is concerned with laboratory blood tests that evaluate renal function. In addition, laboratory values provide information regarding the patient's ability to detect blood clotting disorders. Tests for renal function and clotting ability of blood include prothrombin time (PT), partial thromboplastin time (PTT), platelet (thrombocyte) count, blood urea and nitrogen (BUN), and creatinine levels. The combination of these tests will influence the use of contrast medium, the use of a CT-assisted interventional procedure, or both.

PT is the laboratory test that determines the time required for the formation of clots. Prothrombin is produced by the liver and is a vitamin K–dependent glycoprotein necessary for the formation of a firm fibrin clot. The PT value is reported as the time required for plasma to form a clot, including the time for a laboratory control sample to clot. A value within 2 s of the control sample is considered within a normal range. The normal range for PT in a healthy adult is 10 to 15 s.

PTT is the laboratory test that evaluates the coagulation process for recalcified citrated plasma to clot after partial thromboplastin is added to it. PTT is used to monitor the effectiveness of heparin therapy and to screen for coagulation disorder. The normal adult level of PTT is between 30 and 45 s.

Platelets are the nonnucleated cells that function for clot retraction and coagulation. Platelets are formed by the bone marrow and released into the bloodstream to function in homeostasis. Platelet (thrombocyte) count is the laboratory test for the amount of platelets present in a person's bloodstream. The normal adult level is 150,000/μL to 400,000/μL.

BUN is the concentration of urea or plasma specified in terms of nitrogen content. BUN is an important indication of renal function. BUN can be elevated in disorders that can lead to renal failure. The normal range for BUN is 5 to 20 mg/dL or 1.8 to 7.1 mmol/L. The term azotemia is used in cases for which levels of urea nitrogen are elevated in the bloodstream.

Creatinine is the nitrogenous compound formed as a result of creatine metabolism. Creatinine is formed in muscle in small amounts and is passed into the bloodstream and excreted in the urine. An increased serum creatinine level is an indicator of renal dysfunction. For women, the normal creatinine level is 0.5 to 1.1 mg/dL or 47 to 97 μmol/L. The creatinine level for men is slightly higher. The normal adult male level is 0.6 to 1.2 mg/dL or 53 to 106 μmol/L.

It is the responsibility of the technologist to inform the physician of any laboratory values that are outside the acceptable limit. The examination may need to be canceled or rescheduled until the laboratory values can be returned to the acceptable limits. In the event the laboratory values cannot be stabilized to acceptable limits, the alternative may be to proceed with the CT examination without the use of contrast medium or to use an alternative imaging modality such as MRI or ultrasound.

CT EXPERIENCE REQUIREMENTS FOR PROCEDURES REQUIRING THE SELECTION OF CONTRAST AGENTS, INCLUDING CONTRA-INDICATIONS AND ALLERGY PREPARATION

Mandatory minimum required is 5.

Common Indications

- Demonstration of tumors, lesions, and aneurysm
- Opacification of bowel to allow for the differentiation of normal bowel from lesion

Imaging Considerations

To improve contrast resolution between enhancing structures and nonenhancing structures, the use of contrast medium is used frequently for CT examinations. Contrast agents used in a CT examination can be divided into two main categories of positive and negative contrast agents. Positive contrast agents will attenuate the incoming x-ray photons. The amount of attenuation will determine the intensity of the displayed image. Contrast medium that attenuates a large number of x-ray photons will have a bright or hyperintense appearance. Contrast that allows for the easy passage or reacts in a transparent way will display a dark or hypointense appearance. Structures that are highly attenuating of x-ray photons include bone. Low attenuating structures include lung tissue.

Positive contrast media will provide a hyperintense appearance. An example of a positive contrast agent used in computed tomography is barium sulfate. Negative contrast agents allow the x-ray photons to pass through the structure easier. An example of a negative contrast agent used in computed tomography is air. Air introduced to a patient's stomach will expand the lumen and allow for the demonstration of stomach wall.

Contrast media used in CT procedures can be injected or introduced into the gastrointestinal tract either orally or rectally. The most frequently used type of contrast medium in each of the categories will be discussed. Because there are several trade names, a general description of each type of contrast will be used. The examples contained within the area of contrast medium do not supersede the manufacturer's recommendation or the standards of practice of the imaging facility. The use of contrast medium is similar to other prescribed medications. The success of the procedure is dependent on an accurate patient history, proper administration of medication, and monitoring of the patient's condition after the administration of the medication.

INJECTABLE CONTRAST MEDIUM

Intravenous injections of contrast medium are used to differentiate contrast enhancing structures, such as vascular structure of the brain, from nonenhancing structures. Injectable contrast medium is frequently iodine based. The high atomic number of iodine is responsible for the attenuation of the x-ray photons. Two common choices of injectable contrast medium are ionic and nonionic iodinated contrast agents. The differences of each iodinated contrast agent will be discussed in general because the technologist should always refer to the contrast medium package insert to ascertain the specific chemical information, indications, contraindications, and proper dosage before the product use. A general definition of osmolality and viscosity is necessary as part of the discussion of intravenous contrast medium, because osmolality and viscosity are responsible for many of the undesirable traits of contrast medium.

Osmolality is the total number of particles dissolved per unit of solvent. For example, the osmolality of plasma is 285 milliosmoles per kilogram (mOsm/kg) of water. Ionic contrast medium is 1300 to 1600 mOsm/kg and nonionic contrast medium is 500 to 880 mOsm/kg. The higher osmolality of iodinated contrast medium is considered "hypertonic." The higher osmolality numbers increase the likelihood of negative responses. After the injection of a hypertonic contrast medium, the body tries to maintain homeostasis by allowing a net movement of water into the vascular space. The physical response to this net movement is dehydration; therefore, it is important for the patient to be well hydrated before and after the CT examination requiring the use of iodinated contrast medium.

Viscosity describes the thickness of a fluid. For example, cold syrup has a higher viscosity than hot syrup. The viscosity of ionic contrast medium is 5 to 20 centipoise (cp) at room temperature. Viscosity of iodinated contrast medium can be reduced by warming it before the injection. Combination warming and storage devices are designed to maintain the contrast medium at temperatures comparable to a person's body temperature.

IONIC VS. NONIONIC IODINATED CONTRAST MEDIUM

Ionic iodinated contrast medium has the characteristic of disassociating into ions after injection into the patient. As a result, there is an increase in osmolality for ionic contrast medium when compared with nonionic contrast agents. The viscosity of ionic contrast agents is not significantly different from nonionic agents. Nonionic contrast medium will typically cost three times more, compared with ionic contrast agents. The number of adverse reactions after ionic contrast injections is higher when compared with nonionic agents, especially in patients with a previous reaction to iodine. Differences between ionic and nonionic contrast agents are demonstrated in Table 13-1.

Patients that are hypersensitive to iodine are a contraindication for the use of iodinated contrast medium. The technologist should be aware of the number of other conditions that warrant concern for the patient before the injection of contrast medium. Patients with a functional disorder of the liver or kidneys should not be injected with iodinated contrast medium. Blood urea and nitrogen and creatinine are laboratory tests to determine the functional ability of kidneys. Each contrast manufacturer and imaging facility has an acceptable range of values for BUN and creatinine laboratory tests. These values will include a patient's weight and size. The package insert of the contrast medium will have a complete list of contraindications and warnings for patients who are likely to experience adverse reactions to the

TABLE 13-1

Comparison Between Ionic and Nonionic Iodinated Contrast Media

Ionic Iodinated Contrast	Nonionic Iodinated Contrast
Dissociates/forms ions	Remains intact following injection
Osmolality, 1300–1600 mOsm/kg	Osmolality, 500–850 mOsm/kg
Viscosity, 5–20 cp	Viscosity is not significantly different than ionic contrast agents
Same contraindication as for nonionic contrast agents	Same contraindications as for ionic contrast agents
Cost is approximately ⅓ less than nonionic agents	Cost is approximately 3 times more than ionic agents
Reactions following injections are higher than nonionic agents	Reactions after injections are lower than ionic agents

TABLE 13-2

Common Contraindications for the Use of Injectable Contrast Medium

Hypersensitivity to iodine	Thyrotoxicosis
Functional disturbances of the kidneys	Myelomatosis
Functional disturbances of the liver	Hyperthyroidism
Congestive heart disease	Hay fever
Previous reaction to contrast media	Asthma
Sickle cell disease	Pheochromocytoma
Diabetes	Multiple myeloma
Allergies to food	Anuria

contrast medium. Many facilities will consider the following list as contraindications for the injection of iodinated contrast medium (Table 13-2).

When the benefit of the examination outweighs the risk of allergic reaction to the contrast medium, the physician may choose to medically pretreat the patient before the injection of contrast medium. The premedication regimen is specific to the physician's request. High-risk patients may be administered a corticosteroid, antihistamine, or both, for the pretreatment. The administration process can begin the evening before or immediately before the examination. The use of diazepam has been administered for patients with a history of seizures as a pretreatment method. Diabetic patients may have to alter insulin injection times, amounts, or type of medication to avoid adverse reaction to the contrast medium. The method of pretreatment for contrast reactions is specific for the imaging facility. To completely avoid a reaction to contrast medium, the physician may choose to forgo the use of contrast medium or use another imaging modality such as MRI or ultrasound. The technologist should be familiar with the methods of pretreatment for the imaging facility.

ORAL CONTRAST MEDIUM

Oral contrast medium is frequently based on a dilute solution of barium sulfate ($BaSO_4$) or iodinated contrast medium. Unlike the thick solution of barium sulfate used in the diagnostic radiography, computed tomography typically uses a 1% weight-to-volume diluted version of barium sulfate. Higher concentrations of barium will have a tendency to generate streak artifacts. Iodinated contrast medium is diluted according to the manufacturer's recommendations and the radiologist's preference. Iodinated contrast medium can be diluted with water or juice. A high concentration of iodinated contrast solution will generate streak artifacts during the CT examination. Some physicians will require distention of the patient's stomach during an abdominal CT examination. To provide distention, the patient will ingest the iodinated contrast medium mixed with a carbonated beverage. This method will allow for distention of the gastric wall.

The amount of ingested contrast medium is dependent on the physician's preference and specific area of interest on the CT examination. If the goal of the examination is for the opacification of the entire gastrointestinal tract, the patient will consume contrast medium in intervals before the examination. This process may vary slightly among imaging facilities. If the patient is unable to drink the contrast medium, it may be necessary to administer the contrast solution through a nasogastric tube. When the stomach is the main area of interest, the patient will be required to consume 350 to 500 mL of oral contrast immediately before the examination. Patients scheduled for a CT examination, with the area of interest including the entire small bowel, will need to consume 350 to 500 mL of contrast solution 1 to 2 h before the examination and another 350 to 500 mL immediately before the examination. For complete opacification of the gastrointestinal tract, some physicians require the consumption of 350 to 500 mL of oral contrast medium the evening before or at least 4 to 6 h before the examination. The patient will still need to consume the other doses of contrast medium 1 to 2 h before the examination and the 350 to 500 mL of oral contrast immediately before the examination. This method of contrast consumption will fill the majority of the colon and proximal end of the gastrointestinal tract. Some imaging facilities require the use of a 150- to 250-mL volume of barium solution introduced rectally to opacify the distal portion of the rectum and large bowel.

CONTRAINDICATIONS FOR THE USE OF ORAL CONTRAST MEDIUM

Patients with a known history of hypersensitivity to barium sulfate are a contraindication for the use of barium sulfate. Patients suspected of a perforated bowel should not consume barium sulfate based contrast medium. In the event of a perforated bowel, the contrast medium will spill into the peritoneal cavity. The patient can experience barium peritonitis, which can result in the surgical removal of the barium.

One of the functions of the bowel is for the removal of fluids. When fluids are removed from the barium solution, the patient has the potential for becoming impacted. For this reason, the patient is frequently instructed to consume fluids after the CT examination to prevent barium impaction. If the patient is suffering from colon obstruction, tracheoesophageal fistula, or obstruction lesions of the gastrointestinal tract, the use of barium sulfate for oral contrast medium is contraindicated. An alternative method for the use of barium sulfate is the use of iodinated contrast medium or an alternative diagnostic examination such as MRI or ultrasound.

Patients allergic or sensitive to iodine should not be given iodinated contrast medium. Patients given oral iodinated contrast medium may experience diarrhea, abdominal pain, or flatulence. The concentration of oral iodinated contrast medium is 6 to 9 mg of iodine per milliliter, with total dose ranging from 500 to 1000 mL. Oral contrast medium is a diluted version of iodinated intravenous contrast medium; therefore, the contraindications for oral contrast medium are similar to those of intravenous iodinated contrast medium. If the need for contrast medium supersedes the potential for a reaction, the physician may prescribe a method of pre-examination medication to prevent a reaction to iodinated contrast medium.

CT EXPERIENCE REQUIREMENTS FOR PROCEDURES REQUIRING THE PREPARATION OF CONTRAST AGENTS

Mandatory minimum required is 5.

Common Indications

- Preparation of injectable, oral, and rectally administered contrast agents for the enhancement of contrast absorbing structures

Imaging Considerations

Contrast medium is routinely used as part of the CT examination of the head, chest, abdomen, and pelvis. Many imaging facilities require the patient to understand and sign an agreement for the use of the contrast medium. Most imaging facilities require an interview questionnaire be completed by the technologist and patient before the examination involving the use of contrast medium. Contrast forms should include questions and statements such as the following:

Patient's name

Date of examination

Type of examination

The patient's history of allergies

Allergic reactions to contrast medium

Current use of medications

History of the following:
Diabetes and treatment
Multiple myeloma
Pheochromocytoma
Sickle cell disease
Thyroid disorder

Renal failure

Hay fever

Previous surgeries

Status of pregnancy

Laboratory values of BUN, and creatinine if available

Explanation of complications that may accompany the use of contrast medium

The use of the contrast medium must be within the guidelines of the radiologist and contrast manufacturer recommendations. It is the preference of the radiologist and/or facility to require laboratory tests on the patient before the examination to avoid adverse reactions or any contraindications to the use of the contrast medium. The package insert that accompanies the contrast medium will contain a complete list of information concerning the use and contraindications of the specific contrast agent. The items listed on the package insert include:

Chemical description

Clinical pharmacology

Contraindications

Warnings

Precautions

Adverse reactions

Dosage and administration

Individual indications

Individual usage for contrast agent

The preparation of contrast medium largely depends on the desired effect of the contrast agent. The technologist must be sure that the contrast medium selected is correct for the examination process. As a safety precaution, only contrast medium meant for the specific use in CT examinations should be stored within the computed tomography department. The discussion for contrast preparations is divided into the categories of injectable and orally or rectally applied. The exact preparation of contrast medium is dependent on the imaging facility and contrast manufacturer's recommendations. The technologist should know the location and specifications of contrast mediums within the imaging department.

INJECTABLE CONTRAST MEDIUM

When reading the contrast label, the technologist must be sure that the bottle contains the desired type (ionic vs. nonionic, high vs. low osmolality) of contrast agent. Bottles of injectable contrast medium should be visually inspected before use. Any bottle of contrast medium found to be damaged or left open should be considered contaminated and not be used. Each bottle will have an expiration date displayed. Any bottle found not displaying a date or having an expired date should not be used for injection. If the contrast medium displays an abnormal discoloration or sedimentation, the contrast medium must not be used. Injectable contrast medium should be kept as close to a person's normal body temperature to reduce the viscosity. Certain CT examinations may not require the complete use of a bottle of contrast medium; it is recommended to dispose of the remaining contrast medium after the completion of the examination.

ORAL AND RECTAL CONTRAST MEDIA

Some imaging facilities will use premixed oral contrast medium, whereas other imaging sites prefer to control the concentration of the oral contrast medium. Regardless of the method, the palpability of oral contrast medium can be improved by serving it chilled. Premixed barium based contrast agents have the tendency to "settle"; therefore, it is recommended that the contrast medium be shaken before consumption. Imaging centers that choose to mix the barium or iodinated based contrast, the concentration is determined by the imaging facility. The technologist must exercise caution to prevent an excessive concentration that will result in streak artifacts during the examination. When using iodinated oral contrast medium, the concentration is significantly less than barium solution. The taste of iodinated contrast medium can be improved by mixing it with a flavored drink or juice. This mixing is normally a choice of the imaging facility or radiologist. The technologist may have to administer the oral contrast medium by means of a nasogastric tube in the event that the patient is unable to swallow the oral contrast medium.

Contrast medium may be administered rectally to opacify the distal portion of colon and rectum. A prepared concentration of barium based contrast medium is frequently used for enema administration.

CT EXPERIENCE REQUIREMENTS FOR PROCEDURES REQUIRING THE SITE SELECTION OF AN INTRAVENOUS INJECTION

Mandatory minimum required is 5.

Common Indications

- Minimize the potential for extravasation
- Reduce the possibility of restricted flow of contrast medium caused by patient positioning or previous surgeries
- Reduce the potential for contrast reactions with current drug administration

Imaging Considerations

The use of intravenous contrast medium is routinely used as part of CT examinations of the abdomen, pelvis, and head. Introduction of contrast medium by the use of a bolus injection with single or dual injection rates has become the preferred choice over drip infusion methods. Some imaging sites choose to hand-inject doses of 50 mL or less, whereas other departments prefer the consistency and reproducibility of a power injection system. CT examination of the abdomen and pelvis can require 100 to 200 mL of injectable contrast medium.

The use of a power injector is used routinely as part of the CT examination. Power injectors are programmed by the technologist to deliver the contrast medium at a designated rate and pressure. Reproducibility is a critical advantage of power injection, but at the same time, it requires an additional set of precautions when compared with manual hand injections. For these reasons, the amount of contrast agent and the choice of hand injection instead of power injection methods are determined by the radiologist and imaging facility. The injection site is determined by a combination of factors that include the following:

The contrast manufacturer's recommendations

Imaging facility's standards

The patient's current history and condition

Prior surgeries that can affect the flow of contrast medium

For CT injections the site selection of upper extremities should be chosen over lower extremities except in the case of extreme emergency. Sites commonly selected for the injection of contrast medium include the basilic and cephalic veins of the arms, at the antecubital space. The anastomosis between the basilic and cephalic veins secures the basilic vein from rolling when inserting the catheter or butterfly needle to start the injection site. The basilic and cephalic veins provide an access point for the injection of large amounts of contrast medium. When the arm is extended above the patient's head, the basilic vein is less likely to constrict the flow of contrast medium when compared with the cephalic vein. The technologist should consider the patient's ability to position the arms as part of the site selection process.

Unlike the basilic vein, the dorsal veins of the hand will frequently roll when starting the butterfly needle or catheter. The technologist should provide traction to the skin to stabilize the vein when the needle is inserted. Because of their smaller size, the dorsal veins should be reserved for small-bore catheters with a reduced rate of injection. Injections on the ventral side of the hand and wrist should be avoided because of the location of the radial nerve.

Patients will sometimes arrive at the computed tomography departments with an intravenous site already in place. The technologist cannot assume that the location is suitable for the injection of contrast medium. The technologist should determine the reason the site was chosen and the type of medication used for the current site before deciding whether to use that site for CT contrast injection. Each imaging facility should have a list of standards and protocols for the injection of contrast medium through existing intravenous lines. The contraindications should include the specific medications, patient history, and the compatibility of the contrast medium with the medication. The combination of physician, pharmacist, and package insert from the contrast medium will provide the necessary information and acceptable method of injection through a current intravenous site.

To avoid patient and technical complications, many imaging facilities do not recommend the injection of contrast medium through existing central venous catheters. In cases of recent mastectomy, the technologist should consider the injection of the opposite side. Some CT examinations will dictate site selection, as in the case of a CT examination of the brachial plexus. It is recommended to inject the arm that is contralateral to the side of primary interest to avoid streak artifacts generated from the contrast medium.

Considerations for site selection:

Patient's previous surgeries

Patient's condition

Patient presenting with:

Pre-catheterization

Current medication administration

Current medication going through current site

Type of CT examination

Ability for patient to position after the intravenous site is chosen

CT EXPERIENCE REQUIREMENTS FOR PROCEDURES REQUIRING VENIPUNCTURE

Mandatory minimum required is 5. This procedure may be simulated in those states or institutions where venipuncture by a registered technologist is prohibited.

Common Indications

- Method of quick absorption of medication into the circulatory system
- Method of quick response for medication
- Alternative solution for drugs which cannot be given orally

Imaging Considerations

Intravenous injections are a method of introducing medications or contrast medium into the circulatory system. The response to the medication is rapid and can be the choice of administration when the drug is impalpable or the patient is unable to orally consume the drug. Not all clinical settings allow the registered technologist to start or inject intravenous contrast medium. Registered technologists permitted to inject intravenous drugs should familiarize themselves with facility standards. If the facility does not allow the registered technologist to start the infusion site, the technologist can still assist the qualified personnel by organizing the necessary supplies for starting an infusion site.

It is prudent for the technologist to obtain the patient's vital signs before an intravenous injection. This allows a baseline for comparison in the event of a sudden change to the patient's condition after the injection of drugs or contrast medium. A drug administered intravenously will generate a rapid response; in addition, the drug cannot be retrieved once injected into the person. For these reasons, the technologist should never leave the patient after the administration of an intravenous drug or contrast agent. The patient should be visually and verbally monitored throughout the examination process.

Medical asepsis is mandatory for all drugs and contrast to be administered intravenously. Certain drugs can be given intravenously through an existing intravenous line. This administration is dependent on the following factors:

Facility specification

Type of the pre-existing line

Type of drug present in the existing line

Specific drug to be administered

Amount of drug or contrast to be administered

Rate at which the drug or contrast medium is to be administered

The same factors will determine the type and size of catheter to be used in the event a new intravenous site must be found. Drugs administered slowly or that have low viscosity can be injected through a smaller gauge needle such as a 20- to 25-gauge needle. For drugs that are to be introduced over a long period of time or in large amounts such as 100 to 1000 mL, consider the use of a 20-gauge needle to administer the drug. In addition, the injection of very viscid drugs or contrast medium should consider the use of a larger bore needle. Most facilities prefer the use of a butterfly needle, venous, or angiocatheters to administer drugs or contrast medium. The process and necessary supplies needed for starting an infusion site will vary slightly among facilities; therefore, the technologist should be familiar with the specific protocols (Fig. 13-1). As part of the venipuncture process, the technologist should have all the materials prepared

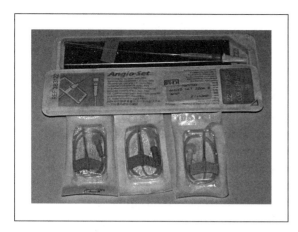

FIGURE 13-1
Different catheters.

before the patient enters in the examination room. In addition to the catheter, other items to prepare include the following items:

Gloves

Tourniquet

Two 3-in. strips of tape

Alcohol or povidone-iodine cleaning pads

Adhesive bandage

Cotton balls

One-piece or multiple-piece catheter

Heparin or buffle cap

10-mL saline solution

10-mL syringe

Before starting the infusion site, the technologist is required to wash his or her hands. Next, the tourniquet should be placed superior to the injection site. The technologist should secure the tourniquet to enhance the appearance of the vein. To increase the diameter of the vein, the patient may be instructed to pump the fist or the technologist may need to briskly "slap" the selected site to dilate the veins. Some situations may require the use of a warm towel wrapped around the selected site to promote dilation of veins. After the tourniquet has been placed and injection site selected, the area should be cleansed with alcohol or a povidone-iodine solution. The cleaning process should be in a circular pattern radiating from the inner to outer area of the site. A 4-in. diameter area should be cleaned at the injection site.

The technologist should wear gloves before inserting the catheter. The vein can be stabilized, by applying a downward pressure and making the skin taut, to the area distal to the insertion site. The bevel of the needle should be placed up, and the catheter should be angled 20° to 45° to the skin. The catheter should be advanced in a smooth consistent motion until the needle tip penetrates the surface of the vein. Blood will return in the catheter tubing as evidence of the vein penetration. Do not extend the catheter through the posterior wall of the vein. If a butterfly-type catheter is used, the angle of insertion should be reduced and inserted 0.25 to 0.05 in. farther into the vein. Release the tourniquet to allow the normal flow of blood through the vein. At this time, the technologist should apply a piece of tape across the butterfly tabs and secure the catheter to the skin to avoid accidentally dislodging the catheter.

When using a two-piece catheter system, once the metal needle portion has penetrated the anterior vein wall, the needle should not be advanced any further. Blood returning into the catheter reservoir portion of the catheter will provide evidence of penetration to the anterior vein wall. At this time, the flexible portion of the catheter should be advanced into the vein while the metal sheath remains stable and acts as a guide for the catheter. The distal portion of the flexible catheter should rest against the patient's skin when fully inserted. At this time, remove the tourniquet to allow the normal flow of blood. The rigid metal needle is now completely removed, and a buffle or heparin cap is secured to the distal end of the flexible catheter. Tape can now be applied across the heparin cap while leaving access to the injection end of the cap. The metal portion of the catheter should be placed in the proper disposal container.

Before the injection of contrast medium, it is advised to test the injection site by administering a small amount of saline. The technologist can inject the saline at a consistent flow while, at the same time, watching for extravasation. If the saline is seen to infiltrate into the subcutaneous tissue, the technologist should stop the injection immediately. After the removal of the catheter, the technologist should apply a warm compress to the site. Notation of the extravasation should be made on the patient's record after the examination process.

The following items should be included on the list of precautions concerning venipuncture:

If an attempt to start an intravenous site is *not* successful, do *not* use the same needle to try another location

If an intravenous site is unsuccessful, the new site should be superior to the previous site

If infiltration of the site occurs, immediately stop the injection and attend to the problem

The following are symptoms of infiltration or extravasation:

Cool skin surrounding the injection site

A burning sensation during the injection

Swelling or redness to the site during injection

To prevent contamination and the introduction of germs to the patient, the technologist should avoid touching any portion of the catheter that will be inserted into the patient.

After the completion of the CT examination, the technologist will remove the catheter before dismissing the patient. Gloves should be worn when removing the catheter from the injection site. The tape should be gently removed from the catheter while leaving the catheter in place. The technologist can now place a cotton ball over the injection site. The catheter can now be removed in consistent smooth motion. When the catheter is removed, the technologist should apply pressure to the cotton ball. Upon removal, the technologist should inspect the catheter for completeness. Constant pressure can be applied to the injection site with manual pressure or by taping the cotton ball to the patient's skin. When the bleeding has stopped, place an adhesive bandage on the injection site. The venipuncture material should be properly disposed of before the technologist washes his or her hands. The technologist should inspect the injection site and instruct the patient for a possible hematoma before dismissing the patient.

CT EXPERIENCE REQUIREMENTS FOR PROCEDURES REQUIRING THE USE OF POWER INJECTORS

Mandatory minimum required is 5.

Common Indications

- Consistent and reproducible method of injection of contrast medium
- Method for injecting a variety of rates and amounts of contrast medium

Imaging Considerations

Mechanical or power injectors are an alternative to hand injection of contrast medium. The power injector provides a reproducible method of injection. The method of injections can vary in the amount and rate of injections. Some CT examinations will require a dual injection rate to provide optimal contrast enhancement of the area of interest. Many of the injectors provide the option of both high and low pressure settings for injections. The injector system includes an actual injection device, injection console, and triggering device.

A simplified explanation of injector mechanics is an electrical motor that drives a threaded rod, which is attached to the piston of the syringe. As the motor turns the rod, the syringe piston advances. The injection console is used to program the rate and amount of contrast to be injected. There are safety devices within the console that provide pressure- and volume-limiting devices. The technologist can

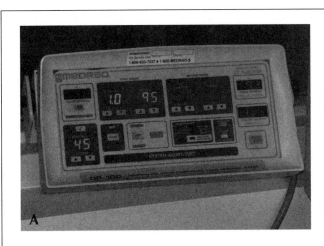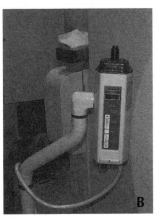

FIGURE 13-2

A: Close-up of console and injector head. B: Contrast injector.

also program the injector rate to initiate the injection rate in a "ramp up" method to avoid a sudden surge of contrast medium at the beginning of the injection. The injection can be manually started from the console or attached to an extension cord which will allow for the close inspection of the injection site during the injection. Some power injectors are designed to inject only when pointed at the floor to allow air to rise to the top of the syringe. Many modern injectors are equipped with an air detection system to avoid the accidental injection of a large bolus of air (Fig. 13-2).

It is not the purpose of this manual to delegate the amounts and rates of injections that should be used for CT examinations. The injection rates, amounts, and delay time between injection and imaging are determined by the radiologist, manufacturer of the injector, CT scanner, and the type of contrast medium used. Many imaging facilities use power injectors for all CT examinations requiring the use of intravenous contrast medium, to provide a consistent and reproducible examination. There are numerous safety features designed in power injection systems, but the safest manner of injection requires the presence of the technologist to visually and physically observe the injection site in the event of extravasation or malfunction of the injection system. The technologist should also be aware of emergency stop devices associated with power injectors. These devices will stop the injection of contrast medium. In the event of extravasation, the injection process should be immediately stopped. The extravasation area should be attended to before proceeding with the examination.

Power injection systems require a specialized syringe for the injection. The syringe is sterilized and disposable for power injectors. Syringe sizes range from 60 to 260 mL in capacity. Extra syringes should be located within the imaging room in the event a syringe is accidentally damaged or contaminated during the loading process.

Disposable syringes should be properly disposed of after the CT examination.

Intravenous contrast medium should be warmed to or near body temperature to reduce the viscosity of solution. Most power injectors have warming bands that are placed around the preloaded syringe. The warming device is used to maintain the syringe and contents at approximately 37°C (98°F). The warming band is designed to maintain the temperature and not for the initial heating of the contrast medium.

When using the power injector, the technologist should assemble all necessary items before the arrival of the patient. The technologist should prepare supplies necessary for venipuncture; disposable injector syringe, flexible tubing, and contrast medium. Upon opening the injector syringe, the technologist should inspect the syringe for any damage. Normally, a rigid filler tube will accompany the syringe container. The plunger of the injector should be withdrawn in the injector before loading the syringe. Place and secure the syringe within the power injector. Aim the injector upward and advance the syringe piston to eliminate the air from the injector syringe. Place the rigid filler tube on the tip of the syringe. The cap and rubber stopper should now be removed from the contrast medium. The opening of the contrast medium bottle is placed over the rigid filler tube. The piston of the syringe should now be returned toward the injector until the contrast has filled the syringe or the desired amount is attained. The rigid filler tube and empty bottle of contrast medium should be disposed of after the CT examination. The filler tube is designed for a single use. In addition, any remaining contrast medium within the bottle should be disposed of and not used for an additional examination. The technologist can now secure the flexible tubing to the contrast injector. The syringe piston should again be advanced to fill the tubing with contrast medium and remove air within the flexible tubing. The end of the flexible tubing is secured to the injector to avoid accidental contamination. The injector is now placed in a downward position to allow any remaining air to rise to the back of the syringe.

CT EXPERIENCE REQUIREMENTS FOR MONITORING PATIENTS FOR ADVERSE REACTIONS

Mandatory minimum required is 5.

Common Indications

- Prevention and assessment of adverse reactions after drug administration during a CT examination

Imaging Considerations

A harmful effect after the administration of a drug is considered an "adverse reaction." When compared with ionic contrast agents, the use of nonionic injectable contrast medium has reduced the amount of adverse reactions. Prophylactic treatment of patients with prior reactions, or a history indicating the potential for a reaction, has also reduced the number of adverse reactions after drug administration. The potential chance for an adverse reaction exists with every patient. Because the computed tomography technologist is present during the injection of contrast agents, it is the technologist's responsibility to monitor the patient for any adverse reaction.

Adverse drug reactions can occur immediately or be delayed after drug administration. Many facilities observe patients for adverse reaction for 30 to 60 min after the injection of contrast medium. Adverse reactions are divided into three categories of mild, moderate, and severe (Table 13-3).

TABLE 13-3

Categories of Adverse Drug Reactions

Mild Adverse Reactions	Moderate Adverse Reactions	Severe Adverse Reactions
Nausea & vomiting	Can have a more pronounced version of mild reactions	Potentially life-threatening: can have a more pronounced version of moderate reactions
Coughing	Changes in pulse	Convulsions
Headache	Bronchospasm	Unresponsiveness
Dizziness	Laryngospasm	Cardiac arrest
Itching	Hyper- or Hypotension	Arrhythmia
Chills	Dyspnea	
Sweats		
Swelling to the eyes and face		
Urticaria		

Treatment of Mild Reactions	Treatment of Moderate Reactions	Treatment of Severe Reactions
Close observation and often no additional treatment	Close observation and often treatment is required but hospitalization is not	Quick observation of symptoms; treatment and hospitalization

Larger doses of contrast medium show an increase in adverse reactions; however, adverse reactions can occur with small doses. Severe reactions occur less frequently than mild reactions. When severe reactions do occur, the CT examination must be stopped, allowing personnel to completely focus on the patient. Severe reactions should be treated in a manner similar to any emergency situation.

Mild reactions require only observation and monitoring of the patient's condition. It should be understood that a mild reaction can accelerate into a severe reaction at any time. A moderate reaction will require treatment and continued observation. When a moderate reaction occurs, the priority of the patient comes before the completion of the CT examination. In the event of a severe adverse reaction, the technologist should stay with the patient and summon assistance along with notification to the radiologist. The technologist should remain calm and continue communication with the patient to gain information regarding the patient's condition and comfort. Any change in the patient's condition should be observed and the time noted. The technologist must be prepared to assist with oxygen, intravenous fluid, and medication administration. As a safety precaution many facilities recommend two qualified personnel present during examinations requiring the injection of contrast agents.

CHAPTER 14

Experience Requirement for the Functions for Image Display

Function	Mandatory	Elective
Geometric measurements	5	
Region of interest	5	
Histograms		3
Highlighting (identify)		3
Target/zoom	5	

CT EXPERIENCE REQUIREMENTS FOR THE USE OF GEOMETRIC MEASUREMENTS

Mandatory minimum required is 5.

Common Indications

- Measurement of abnormal structures for comparison of dimensions with normal anatomy
- Measurement to determine the approximate volume or size of cystic structures before biopsy procedures

Imaging Considerations

After completion of the CT examination, the technologist may find it necessary to determine the size of abnormal structures as in the case of a hematoma or mass within the liver. The use of geometric measurements is also helpful in determining the size of an aortic aneurysm. CT scanners are equipped with a software package that allows the technologist to take multiple measurements of an area of interest. The different measurements are displayed on the image and can be filmed with the measurements demonstrated on the image. Measurements will be displayed in millimeters or centimeters. Measurements should be taken on areas of interest before a biopsy, drainage, or aspiration procedure.

The technologist activates the measurement software and places the cursor over the border of the area of interest. The first location is

181

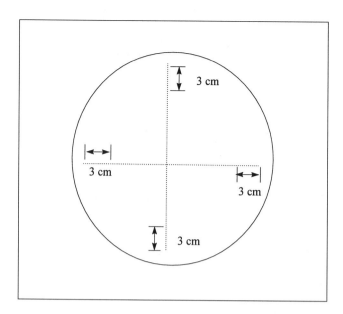

FIGURE 14-1

A measurement grid.

"set," and the cursor is next placed on the opposite border and again set. The measurement will then be displayed on the image. Image measurement uses image data; therefore, measurements can be completed on any image stored on the computer files.

Each CT image is displayed with a reference scale on the side of the image. If the images have already been filmed, the technologist can use a ruler in conjunction with the reference scale. This method will enable the technologist or radiologist to attain an approximate measurement over the area of interest. The technologist should be proficient in both methods of measurement. Quality assurance testing should be performed to verify the accuracy of the measurement device. This testing can be completed by scanning a phantom device with a grid established in the x and y axes. The grid consists of a line of holes in the midhorizontal and midvertical planes of the phantom. The distance measured should be consistent and form the periphery of the phantom. The distances between the grid locations are known and should be compared with the software measurement device (Fig. 14-1).

CT EXPERIENCE REQUIREMENTS FOR THE PROFICIENT DEMONSTRATION OF REGION OF INTEREST SOFTWARE

Mandatory minimum required is 5.

Common Indications

- Determining the statistical calculations that exist within a defined area of anatomy

- A rapid method for determining the density of a specific structure on an image

Imaging Considerations

Region of interest (ROI) is a postprocessing function. The process begins when the technologist determines the area of interest. Once the ROI software is activated, the typical shape of a circle or ellipse will be displayed on the monitor. The shape can vary with scanners and can also be drawn in a free-style manner around irregular objects of interest.

The ROI will calculate and display the average attenuation values that exist within the ROI. The mean attenuation values will be displayed in Hounsfield units (HU). The ROI function will also display the standard deviation within the area of interest. The standard deviation will be a value of zero (0) or higher. If the mean value within a ROI is 90 HU and the standard deviation is 0, this means that all pixels within the ROI have the value of 90; therefore, the area within the ROI is homogenous. If the standard deviation demonstrates a value of 40 with the mean still being 90 HU, there is a variety of attenuation values within the ROI. The larger the standard deviation, the larger the variety of attenuation values within the ROI.

It is important for the technologist not to select any unnecessary areas or use an ROI any larger than necessary. For example, when using the ROI function within a lesion, the technologist should use a small enough ROI to avoid including normal or border tissue in the attenuation calculations. The mean value and standard deviation will be erroneous if the ROI is placed incorrectly.

Another method for finding the attenuation value is also to place the cursor over an area of interest. This method will only display the Hounsfield unit for the pixel beneath the cursor location. The technologist also has other options available once the ROI is selected. These options include image magnification and distance measurement. Some ROI software will allow the transfer of the demonstrated location to the next slice image. The technologist should demonstrate proficiency in all the ROI functions available for the specific CT scanner.

CT EXPERIENCE REQUIREMENTS FOR THE PROFICIENT DEMONSTRATION OF HISTOGRAM SOFTWARE

Elective minimum required is 3.

Common Indications

- Demonstration of the frequency of attenuation values within a region of interest

Imaging Considerations

A histogram is displayed as a bar graph representing the frequency of Hounsfield values within a designated ROI. To use the histogram function, the technologist must first determine the area of interest. Activating the histogram function will display a bar graph superimposed on the same CT image on the monitor. The technologist will often perform the histogram function as part of the ROI process.

CT EXPERIENCE REQUIREMENTS FOR THE PROFICIENT DEMONSTRATION OF HIGHLIGHTING SOFTWARE

Elective minimum required is 3.

Common Indications

- A method to determine the average attenuation value within an area of interest by adjusting the level until the maximal number of pixels are highlighted

Imaging Considerations

The highlighting software function demonstrates pixels within an area of interest brighter or more hyperintense than normal. The technologist selects a range of CT attenuation values by using the window and level selections to be highlighted. The resulting product will increase the brightness appearance of the area selected. Highlighting is a method to determine the average attenuation value within an area of interest by adjusting the level until the maximal number of pixels are highlighted to the desired intensity.

CT EXPERIENCE REQUIREMENTS FOR THE PROFICIENT DEMONSTRATION OF TARGET/ZOOM SOFTWARE

Mandatory minimum required is 5.

Common Indications

- A method to increase the diagnostic value of a CT image by using a specific amount of raw data to construct the image

Imaging Considerations

The technologist will frequently use the "Zoom or Targeting" function when performing a CT scan of the lumbar spine. The entire area of the abdomen is scanned and is demonstrated on the first image slice. The technologist and radiologist are only interested in displaying the areas of the spine to include the aorta anteriorly and the posterior and transverse processes of the spine. To do this, the technologist selects a new display field of view to include only this area. The computer will use only the information within the area of interest to construct the image. The next image of the spine will now appear larger because the display field of view only includes the area of the spine. Decreasing the display field of view will increase the appearance of the image size. The technologist should scan a patient with the appropriate field of view to maintain the spatial resolution of the image.

Zoom or targeting should not be confused with magnification. Zoom uses a specific amount of raw data to construct the image. Magnification uses image data that increase the size of the pixels within an area of interest. Magnification does *not* improve spatial resolution. Magnification increases the pixel size without increasing the amount of information within the pixel. Spatial resolution is improved by either reducing the slice thickness, field of view, or both. Another method of improving spatial resolution is by increasing the number of pixels within the matrix. Magnification simply increases the pixel size and, therefore, decreases the resulting spatial resolution. If the image appears too small, the display field of view should be decreased. If the technologist is required to increase the size of images on a previous CT examination, the raw data should be used for the change in the display field of view. However, if image data are the only information available on the previous CT examination, the magnification process may need to be considered.

CHAPTER 15

Experience Requirement for Performing the Quality Assurance Procedures With the Appropriate Phantoms

Procedure	Mandatory	Elective
Calibration (e.g., air, water)	5	
CT number	5	
Noise	5	
Linearity		3
Spatial resolution		3
Contrast resolution		3

CT EXPERIENCE REQUIREMENTS FOR THE PROFICIENT PERFORMANCE OF QUALITY ASSURANCE PROCEDURES CONCERNING CALIBRATION

Mandatory minimum required is 5.

Common Indications

- A quality control method for the calibration of detectors to air and water

Imaging Considerations

There are a variety of quality tests designed to ensure that the optimal CT image is consistently produced. The frequency of these tests will typically depend on the manufacturer's recommendations for the specific test. The frequency of quality tests range from daily to annually. Many scanners provide a method for calibrating the detectors on a daily basis. This quality test is performed by the technologist as part of the daily warm-up regime. Rigorous quality tests will be performed by the factory representative or by the trained personnel employed by the imaging facility.

Performance of quality tests should be consistent with the technical factors and approximate time in completing the test. Cataloging the test result is a vital part of quality testing because changes within the system's quality can be subtle or quick. With consistent record keeping, the technologist can identify changes and address recalibration or service calls in an efficient manner.

The exact technical factors used to perform quality tests are dependent on the CT scanner. Many scanners are designed to use the same technical factors for scanning a head when performing calibration tests. The factors used for a specific quality test should be consistent for the specific test. This method simplifies the process of monitoring changes with test results. The acceptable limits are determined by a range of values that most frequently occur when the scanner is operating optimally. During the initial set-up process of a new CT scanner, the manufacturer's representative will program the technical factors for many of the quality tests. Quality tests are performed periodically and after the replacement of major components such as the x-ray tube or service adjustments.

Most modern CT scanners are designed to perform a "quick calibration test." This quality test is performed as part of the daily start-up procedure for the CT technologist. The quick calibration test may vary slightly among manufacturers, but in general it includes a low technical factor to allow for x-ray tube warm-up. After the warm-up procedure, the x-ray tube and detectors are tested for calibration to air. This process allows the x-ray tube to radiate the detectors with only the attenuation process occurring with the air present in the gantry. The detectors are calibrated to accept the information from the x-ray photons. The goal is for the detectors to produce an image that is homogenous to the incoming x-ray photons.

Some manufacturers recommend a quality test using a water-filled Lucite phantom. The phantom is attached to the head end of the examination table. The phantom has centering marks that provide consistent positioning in the x, y, and z axes of the examination table. Once the phantom is centered, the calibration process is started. The table will retract and remove the phantom from the gantry location and the tube warm-up will begin. After completion of the tube warm-up, the calibration of detectors will continue. The computer will reposition the phantom into the gantry after the calibration of detectors is completed. The water-filled phantom will be imaged and the statistical information will be displayed. Each manufacturer will provide a set of quality guidelines specific for the CT scanner.

CT EXPERIENCE REQUIREMENTS FOR THE PROFICIENT PERFORMANCE OF QUALITY ASSURANCE PROCEDURES CONCERNING THE AREA OF CT NUMBERS

Mandatory minimum required is 5.

Common Indications

- A quality control method for monitoring the consistent production of CT values based on the comparison of water and air

Imaging Considerations

There are a variety of quality tests designed to ensure that the optimal CT image is produced consistently. The frequency of these tests will typically depend on the manufacturer recommendations for the specific test. The frequency of quality tests range from daily to annually. Many scanners provide a method for calibrating the detectors on a daily basis. This quality test is performed by the technologist as part of the daily warm-up regimen. Rigorous quality tests will be performed by the factory representative or by the trained personnel employed by the imaging facility.

Performance of quality tests should be consistent with the technical factors and approximate time in completing the test. Cataloging the test result is a vital part of quality testing because changes within the system's quality can be subtle or quick. With consistent record keeping, the technologist can identify changes and address recalibration or service calls in an efficient manner.

The exact technical factors used to perform quality tests are dependent on the CT scanner. Many scanners are designed to use the same technical factors for scanning a head when performing calibration tests. The factors used for a specific quality test should be consistent for the specific test. This method simplifies the process of monitoring changes with test results. The acceptable limits are determined by a range of values that most frequently occur when the scanner is operating optimally. During the initial set-up process of a new CT scanner, the manufacturer's representative will program the technical factors for many of the quality tests. Quality tests are performed periodically and after the replacement of major components such as the x-ray tube or service adjustments.

Water and air are the two media used for calibration points for CT numbers. A water phantom is used for a variety of quality tests. The manner in which the quality test is performed varies with the specific type of CT scanner. Many scanners require the technologist to attach and center the phantom to the examination table. The phantom is scanned, and the necessary information is automatically displayed and

189

stored within the computer. It is still a necessary part of the technologist's responsibilities to monitor the results to make sure the image quality stays within the acceptable limits. Certain CT scanners will require the technologist to complete the quality tests manually and monitor the acceptable levels. The manual method of performing the CT numbers calibration test will now be discussed.

The water phantom test uses a cylindrical plastic device that measures approximately 20 cm in diameter. Each water phantom will be specific for the type of CT scanner. The phantom is attached to the head of the imaging couch. The cylinder has centering marks for proper positioning and alignment. Centering marks provide consistency in the testing procedure. The phantom is advanced and scanned with the appropriate technical factors. When the image is reconstructed and displayed on the monitor, the technologist can place the region of interest (ROI) in the center of the image. The ROI should be approximately 2 to 3 cm in diameter or include 200 to 300 pixels within the ROI.

The mean value within the ROI is expected to read zero, "0." The acceptable limits of the water phantom test should be 3 Hounsfield units (HU) on either side of 0. Anything outside the ±3 range is unacceptable and may require recalibration of the reconstruction algorithm. This recalibration process is described by certain CT manufacturers for the technologist to perform, or it may require notification to a qualified repair personnel.

The standard deviation can be determined with the same image for testing the mean attenuation value of water. An ideal standard deviation for water would be 0. This would indicate that each pixel within the ROI would demonstrate a value of 0. When using a water phantom, the typical standard deviation values are between 2 HU and 7 HU. As the standard deviation increases, the resulting CT image will demonstrate a "noisier" appearance because the variety of CT numbers increases.

To test the CT values for air, the technologist can place the ROI in an area to include air only. The expected CT number is −1000. The acceptable range of values is 5 HUs on either side of the −1000 HU. If the results of this test are outside the acceptable limits, it may be necessary to recalibrate the algorithm or contact a qualified repair person. The values of mean, standard deviation, and air are dependent on the technical factors, phantom, and the reconstruction algorithm. The proper placement and size of ROI can also influence the results of the quality test.

CT EXPERIENCE REQUIREMENTS FOR THE PROFICIENT PERFORMANCE OF QUALITY ASSURANCE PROCEDURES CONCERNING IMAGE NOISE

Mandatory requirement of 5.

Common Indications

- A quality control method for monitoring the consistent production of CT images with an acceptable amount of noise present

Imaging Considerations

There are a variety of quality tests designed to ensure that the optimal CT image is consistently produced. The frequency of these tests will typically depend on the manufacturer's recommendations for the specific test. The frequency of quality tests range from daily to annually. Many scanners provide a method for calibrating the detectors on a daily basis. This quality test is performed by the technologist as part of the daily warm-up regime. Rigorous quality tests will be performed by the factory representative or by the trained personnel employed by the imaging facility.

Performance of quality tests should be consistent with the technical factors and approximate time in completing the test. Cataloging the test result is a vital part of quality testing, because changes within the system's quality can be subtle or quick. With consistent record keeping, the technologist can identify changes and address recalibration or service calls in an efficient manner.

The exact technical factors used to perform quality tests are dependent on the CT scanner. Many scanners are designed to use the same technical factors for scanning a head when performing calibration tests. The factors used for a specific quality test should be consistent for the specific test. This method simplifies the process of monitoring changes with test results. The acceptable limits are determined by a range of values that most frequently occur when the scanner is operating optimally. During the initial set-up process of a new CT scanner, the manufacturer's representative will program the technical factors for many of the quality tests. Quality tests are performed periodically and after the replacement of major components such as the x-ray tube or service adjustments.

Noise demonstrated in a CT image is a random variation of CT numbers or Hounsfield units when obtained from a known uniform object. Noise will characteristically be displayed as a salt and pepper appearance or grainy image. The variance in Hounsfield units or CT numbers are typically used to quantify noise. Factors such as type of CT scanner, patient size, slice thickness, size of matrix, field of view, convolution filter, and number of detected photons all affect the amount of noise within an image. The acceptable levels of noise are determined by the manufacturer of the CT scanner. Testing for noise is performed on an annual basis.

A 20-cm Lucite water phantom is used to determine the quantity of noise. The phantom is attached and centered to the CT scanner. The phantom is scanned to produce one cross-sectional image. This process is repeated several times with increasing mA settings and slice thicknesses. When scanning the different slices, all other technical factors should remain constant.

The ROI is activated and placed in the middle of the image. The ROI needs to be approximately 2 to 3 cm in diameter or cover 200 to 300 pixels within the ROI. The standard deviation values are determined from the ROI. The expected mean CT value for the water phantom would be "0" HU. The ideal standard deviation would also be zero, "0." A standard deviation of "0" means every pixel within the ROI would have a value of 0 HU. This would suggest the variance of Hounsfield values would be zero from the acceptable value of water, and the medium is homogenous. In reality, noise is also displayed in the cross-sectional image, and the noise will be represented by the value of the standard deviation. The higher the value of standard deviation, the more noise present within the ROI.

The standard deviation will normally decrease in the images with an increase in slice thickness and mA settings. Noise is reduced because more information is present in the thicker slices with a higher mA setting when compared with the thin slices. Noise is divided into the categories of photon and electronic noise. Photon noise occurs because of the lack of photons captured by the detector elements. Electronic noise is an inherent part of the electrical components of the amplifiers, which increase the detected signal. The amount of noise should not increase with age of the CT scanner.

CT EXPERIENCE REQUIREMENTS FOR THE PROFICIENT PERFORMANCE OF QUALITY ASSURANCE PROCEDURES CONCERNING LINEARITY

Elective requirement of 3.

Common Indications

- A quality control method for monitoring the relationship of CT numbers and the linear attenuation of a known material

Imaging Considerations

There are a variety of quality tests designed to ensure that the optimal CT image is consistently produced. The frequency of these tests will typically depend on the manufacturer's recommendations for the specific test. The frequency of quality tests range from daily to annually. Many scanners provide a method for calibrating the detectors on a daily basis. This quality test is performed by the technologist as part of the daily warm-up regime. Rigorous quality tests will be performed by the factory representative or by the trained personnel employed by the imaging facility.

Performance of quality tests should be consistent with the technical factors and approximate time in completing the test. Cataloging the test result is also a vital part of quality testing because changes within the system's quality can be subtle or quick. With consistent record keeping, the technologist can identify changes and address recalibration or service calls in an efficient manner.

The exact technical factors used to perform quality tests are dependent on the CT scanner. Many scanners are designed to use the same technical factors for scanning a head when performing calibration tests. The factors used for a specific quality test should be consistent for the specific test. This method simplifies the process of monitoring changes with test results. The acceptable limits are determined by a range of values that most frequently occur when the scanner is operating optimally. During the initial set-up process of a new CT scanner, the manufacturer's representative will program the technical factors for many of the quality tests. Quality tests are performed periodically and after the replacement of major components such as the x-ray tube or service adjustments.

As the x-ray photons enter a patient, they begin to attenuate. The difference in tissues will cause the amount of attenuation to vary. The amount the photons attenuated per unit of length is referred to as the linear attenuation coefficient. The x-ray beam is polyenergetic; therefore, as the beam proceeds through the tissue, the attenuation process occurs at differing rates. The lower energy x-ray photons are absorbed first, as the beam progresses through the tissue. Attenuation of a polyenergetic x-ray beam will increase the average energy. The term "effective energy" is used when discussing the energy of a polychromatic x-ray beam. The amount of attenuation that occurs is highly dependent on the effective energy of the x-ray photons within the beam.

Linearity is the relationship between CT numbers and the linear attenuation coefficient of a specific substance. The same water phantom is used for the quality test, because the CT numbers of water and the Lucite phantom are known values. "The mean CT values of the water can be plotted as a function of the attenuation coefficients of the phantom materials" (Seeram, 1994). The resulting relationship should be a straight line display, demonstrating an increase in the mean CT number with an increase in the linear attenuation coefficient.

CT EXPERIENCE REQUIREMENTS FOR THE PROFICIENT PERFORMANCE OF QUALITY ASSURANCE PROCEDURES CONCERNING THE AREA OF SPATIAL RESOLUTION

Elective requirement of 3.

Common Indications

- A quality control method for monitoring the spatial resolution of the CT scanner

Imaging Considerations

There are a variety of quality tests designed to ensure the optimal CT image is consistently produced. The frequency of these tests will typically depend on the manufacturer's recommendations for the specific test. The frequency of quality tests range from daily to annually. Many scanners provide a method for calibrating the detectors on a daily basis. This quality test is performed by the technologist as part of the daily warm-up regime. Rigorous quality tests will be performed by the factory representative or by the trained personnel employed by the imaging facility.

Performance of quality tests should be consistent with the technical factors and approximate time in completing the test. Cataloging the test result is a vital part of quality testing, because changes within the system's quality can be subtle or quick. With consistent record keeping, the technologist can identify changes and address recalibration or service calls in an efficient manner.

The exact technical factors used to perform quality tests are dependent on the CT scanner. Many scanners are designed to use the same technical factors for scanning a head when performing calibration tests. The factors used for a specific quality test should be consistent for the specific test. This method simplifies the process of monitoring changes with test results. The acceptable limits are determined by a range of values that most frequently occur when the scanner is operating optimally. During the initial set-up process of a new CT scanner, the manufacturer's representative will program the technical factors for many of the quality tests. Quality tests are performed periodically and after the replacement of major components such as the x-ray tube or service adjustments.

The exact technical factors used to perform a spatial resolution test are dependent on the CT scanner. Factors that affect spatial resolution are field of view, matrix, and slice thickness. The best spatial resolution results from an image with the smallest field of view, highest matrix, and thinnest slice thickness. Technical factors used for a specific quality test should be consistent each time for the same test. This method simplifies the process of monitoring changes with test results. The acceptable limits are determined by the manufacturer of the specific model of scanner. During the initial set-up process of a new CT scanner, the manufacturer's representative will program the technical factors for many of the quality tests.

Spatial resolution is the ability to clearly depict a small object as an individual structure without blurring or distortion from the background of the image. Many CT scanners have a spatial resolution from 0.5 to 1.0 mm. The evaluation of spatial resolution is tested with a line-pair phantom. The phantom contains five small holes filled with water to provide a high contrast appearance. The holes are demonstrated on the phantom lengthwise to give the appearance of a line. There are a series of five holes drilled in a row with a spacing between them that is equal to the diameter of the hole. The next row will contain another series of holes but slightly smaller in diameter and spacing. The row that can be clearly displayed with the smallest holes and spacing demonstrates the best spatial resolution at the time of the scan.

Spatial resolution is measured in millimeter units; however, when the line-pair phantom is used, the value is in line-pairs per centimeter. One hole and one space constitute one line-pair. When the phantom is scanned and the technologist can clearly visualize 10 line-pairs per centimeter, the technologist can divide the 10 millimeters (1 cm) by 20 (10 lines and 10 spaces) and determine the spatial resolution of the CT scanner to be 0.5 mm.

CT EXPERIENCE REQUIREMENTS FOR THE PROFICIENT PERFORMANCE OF QUALITY ASSURANCE PROCEDURES CONCERNING THE AREA OF CONTRAST RESOLUTION

Elective requirement of 3.

Common Indications

- A quality control method for monitoring the contrast resolution of CT images

Imaging Considerations

There are a variety of quality tests designed to ensure the optimal CT image is consistently produced. The frequency of these tests will typically depend on the manufacturer's recommendations for the specific test. The frequency of quality tests range from daily to annually. Many scanners provide a method for calibrating the detectors on a daily basis. This quality test is performed by the technologist as part of the daily warm-up regime. Rigorous quality tests will be performed by the factory representative or by the trained personnel employed by the imaging facility.

Performance of quality tests should be consistent with the technical factors and approximate time in completing the test. Cataloging the test result is a vital part of quality testing, because changes within the system's quality can be subtle or quick. With consistent record keeping, the technologist can identify changes and address recalibration or service calls in an efficient manner.

The exact technical factors used to perform quality tests are dependent on the CT scanner. Many scanners are designed to use the same technical factors for scanning a head when performing calibration tests. The factors used for a specific quality test should be consistent for the specific test. This method simplifies the process of monitoring changes with test results. The acceptable limits are determined by a range of values that most frequently occur when the scanner is operating optimally. During the initial set-up process of a new CT scanner, the manufacturer's representative will program the technical factors for many of the quality tests. Quality tests are performed periodically and after the replacement of major components such as the x-ray tube or service adjustments.

Contrast resolution is the ability to depict subtle differences in densities. The density differences are represented with differing shades of gray. CT scanners can depict 0.5% differences in densities of tissues. This compares to conventional radiography being able to discriminate a 10% difference in densities. Contrast resolution can be determined quantitatively by knowing the linear attenuation coefficient of the x-ray photon as it passes through the phantom and the linear attenuation coefficient of water. The linear attenuation coefficient is a necessary component for determining contrast; it is vital that the technologist use the same kilovolt peak consistently when performing this test. Contrast resolution is also affected by the spatial resolution of the scanner, noise, and visual perception. Any item that affects these factors will also affect the contrast resolution of the CT scanner. The quality test to determine contrast resolution should be performed monthly.

The phantom is affixed to the CT couch and positioned at the proper location within the scanner. The technical factors will influence the success or reliability of this test. The technologist must be faithful at performing this test under consistent conditions. The quality phantom is constructed of Lucite and cylindrical in shape. The phantom contains a series of fluid-filled holes to demonstrate a subtle difference from the surrounding tissue. The holes are in rows forming a radiating pattern, similar to the numbers on the face of a clock. Each row will have holes of the same diameter. As the rows progress in a clockwise pattern, the holes become progressively smaller. When scanned, the phantom will display a cross-section of the cylinder with holes. The image should be displayed with a narrow window width to demonstrate a high contrast difference between the holes and the surrounding matter. Because the x-ray photons attenuate when they pass through the phantom, the contrast difference becomes more subtle.

The purpose of this test is to determine the smallest row of holes that can be "clearly" visualized at the specific technical factors. For many CT scanners, the technologist should be able to visualize the row of holes measuring 4 mm to 5 mm in diameter or smaller. Visualization of the 4-mm to 5-mm row of holes will enable the technologist to depict a 0.5% contrast difference in objects. There should not be an increase in contrast resolution over the life of the scanner. Reduced levels of contrast resolution occur because of the increase in image noise. Image noise increases because of a decrease in mAs or any factor affecting the reduction of x-ray production. Electronic noise is also present because of amplification or noise generated by the x-ray detectors. The importance of this test is based on the comparison of previous tests or manufacturer's standards.

PART 2

MR Imaging Procedures

TECHNOLOGIST ASSURANCES FOR MRI

CHAPTER 16

Pre-Examination Preparations

It has been said the success of the examination has been determined before the first image ever appears on the monitor. The successful completion of the examination can be subdivided into three categories (Table 16-1). The first category falls under the area of pre-examination preparation. Items in this category include a firm understanding of MRI safety procedures, preparation of examination room, selection of the proper protocol, parameters, selection of the optimal imaging coil, and universal precautions. Once the patient has arrived, the second category, that of patient care, is initiated. Patient care actually occurs before, during, and after the examination; however, in this category, the major emphasis is on the patient. The patient-care category includes identification of the patient; safety screening and patient education concerning the procedure; evaluation of requisition, medical record, or both; documentation of patient history, including allergies; patient assessment; documentation of procedure; and patient data in appropriate records. During the imaging process, the images must be of optimal quality. After the imaging process, the technologist must discharge the patient and inform the patient of any postprocedural instructions. The final category of examination imaging includes image display, image filming, and archiving; optimal image quality, including optimal demonstration of anatomic region; proper identification and patient data on images, and examination completeness. It should be understood the three categories are interdependent of one another. At times, each category will blend with the next and, at times, will overlap the adjacent category. The items in each category have no set order, but should be considered as an overall approach to successful completion of the examination. The following pages will cover each category in more depth. All three categories are a critical portion of each MR imaging procedure.

TABLE 16-1

Categories of a Successful MR Imaging Procedure

Pre-examination preparation

MRI safety procedures

Examination room preparation

Selection of proper protocol

Selection of optimal imaging coil

Patient care

Identification of the patient and evaluation of requisition, medical record, or both

Safety screening and patient education concerning the procedure

Documentation of patient history, including allergies

Patient assessment

Patient positioning

Documentation of procedure and patient data in appropriate records

Discharge the patient and inform the patient of any postprocedural instructions

Universal precautions

Examination imaging

Image display, filming, and archiving

Optimal image quality, including demonstration of anatomic region

Proper identification and patient data on images

Examination completeness

Before the technologist can be considered competent, the technologist must be proficient in all three categories on every examination.

MRI examinations start long before the patient arrives at the MRI department. This portion of the examination process deals with the pre-examination preparations necessary to ensure the efficiency of the examination.

MRI SAFETY PROCEDURES

The MRI unit is a controlled environment to ensure the protection of the technologist, ancillary staff, and public. This process is completed by using warning signs and security systems before entering the MR unit itself. MR personnel and ancillary staff should be informed through in-services or other training methods to ensure the necessary safety when working in the atmosphere of an MR unit. It is also wise to use the public relations department within the imaging facility to enhance the public awareness of MRI safety.

No biological effects have been determined from the static magnetic fields generated from diagnostic MR units. Safety precautions include the presence of any electrical, magnetic, or mechanically activated implants in any person intending to be in the proximity of the MR unit. The risk of malfunction of the implant is increased with the influences of the static magnetic field. MRI is currently a contraindication for any person with a cardiac pacemaker. Concerns involving the actual biological effects on a pregnant technologist have been studied, and as a precaution, the technologist should not be in the examination room during image acquisitions. This process is especially important during the first trimester of pregnancy.

The largest threat to personnel working within the MR unit is not from biological considerations but instead from the risk of ferromagnetic projectiles brought within the MR unit itself. Ferromagnetic objects can reach a velocity of 40 mph when affected by the static magnetic field. Regardless of size, the ferromagnetic object can be influenced by the magnetic field of the MR unit. The MR technologist should be watchful for the untrained person bringing items such as an oxygen tank, wheel chair, or pair of hemostats or scissors into the MR unit.

Persons planning on entering the MR unit need to be educated about ferromagnetic material such as oxygen tanks, carts, IV poles, and chairs. This education includes all ancillary personnel. In situations of a code, the patient should be removed from the MR unit before treatment. People associated with fire fighting and law enforcement should also be informed of the necessary measurements involving MR safety. Most fires within the MR unit are electrical in nature; therefore, it is important to understand that turning off the electricity from the MR electrical components will not quickly remove the magnetic effects from a super-conducting or permanent MR magnet. This enlightens the importance of nonferromagnetic fire-fighting equipment. In the event of a fire, all persons should be evacuated from the MR unit as quickly as possible.

The topic of MR safety would not be complete without discussion of an MR quench. An MR quench is the sudden heating and expansion of the cryogen as it changes from a liquid to a gaseous state. A quench can result from the initial ramping-up process to secure the magnets full strength, when the cryogen of liquid helium is being replenished, or if a large ferromagnetic object has attached itself to the side of the magnet. The MR unit is designed to ventilate the liquid helium to the outside in the event of a quench. The risk involved with a quench is suffocation, frostbite, or both, to the patient and staff.

PREPARATION OF EXAMINATION ROOM

First impressions are always important, and the preparation of the MR examination room is no different. The first thing the technologist sees in the morning is the work atmosphere. It is important to have all imaging coils, quality phantoms, and the overall appearance of the work area organized for efficiency. Consistent placement of imaging items will improve the effectiveness of the technologist. First impres-

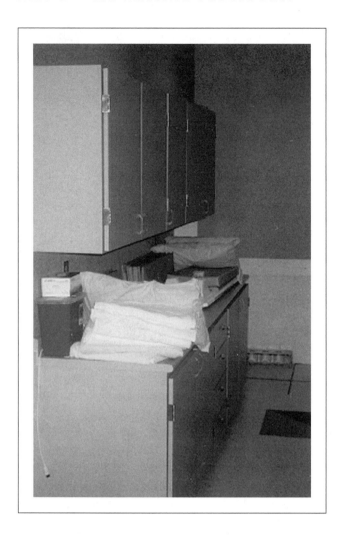

FIGURE 16-1
Cluttered cabinets.

sions are also important for the patient. The patient is often coming into an unfamiliar atmosphere when entering an MRI facility. The easiest judgment comes by visually inspecting the MR department. The technologist and room that appear organized and efficient go toward retaining or improving the confidence of the patient. Before bringing the patient into the imaging room, it is wise for the technologist to have the room organized, including the proper imaging coil either attached to the MR unit or placed in a convenient location for the technologist when positioning the patient (Fig. 16-1).

SELECTION OF PROPER PROTOCOL

The proper selection of protocol is a combined effort between the radiologist, technologist, and manufacturer's requirements. The selection of pulse sequence is based on conventional spin echo and gradient echo imaging. The proper imaging sequence is a combination of acquiring the highest quality image in the least amount of time. This combination is dependent on the patient condition. When selecting a protocol, technologists should ask themselves: "Will the patient be able to tolerate the longer imaging sequence to attain the higher signal image? Does the patient's condition justify a reduction in image quality to trade for a faster scanning time?" These questions rely on the radiologist's and MR technologist's previous experiences.

In addition to patient considerations, the diagnostic considerations are a vital part in selecting the optimal imaging protocol. When selecting the proper protocol, it is important to place consideration to the pulse sequence that will provide the optimal image quality. If the demonstration is for normal anatomy or for the visualization of a pathologic condition, it is important to select the optimal pulse sequence and imaging parameters. In this case, the proper pulse sequence will determine the image weighting and contrast characteristics of the image. The proper protocol selection will place consideration to the anatomy of interest and anatomy that can generate artifacts. These artifacts include flow artifacts from cerebrospinal fluid or blood, artifacts from high lipid areas, and artifacts from both voluntary and involuntary motion. Therefore, the proper protocol involves considerations to patients, specific anatomy, image contrast, and generation of artifacts. As with many diagnostic modalities, selection of the best protocol is a combination of balance and trade-offs between the needs of the patient, technologist, and radiologist.

SELECTION OF PROPER PARAMETERS

Imaging parameters are often the responsibilities of the manufacturer, technologist, and radiologist. Four main factors should be considered when determining image quality. These considerations are signal to noise ratio, contrast to noise ratio, spatial resolution, and scan time. Often, the improvement in one area will result in a degradation to one of the other parameters.

Signal to noise ratio (SNR) is the amount of usable MR signal in relationship to the amount of noise present while generating the signal. The noise of the MR system is inherent electrical noise of the MR system components and noise generated when the patient is placed within the bore of the MR unit. Noise is present with every examination and can vary with the area being imaged. The amount of signal can be fluctuated relative to noise. Increasing the generated signal, therefore, will increase the SNR of the image. Factors that increase the SNR are proton density of the area being imaged, increasing slice thickness, increasing the number of acquisitions to create the image, decreasing the receive bandwidth, use of the proper imaging coil, and use of the proper repetition time (TR), echo time (TE), and flip angles.

Contrast is the difference between shades of gray in an image. Contrast to noise ratio (CNR) is the different shades of gray and are the result of differing signal amplitudes from the generated echoes. Therefore, items that affect signal amplitude will affect CNR. Items that determine contrast of an MR image include TR, TE, TI (inversion time), flip angle, flow, T1, T2, and proton density of the area being scanned.

Spatial resolution is the ability to distinguish two separate points of interest as two independent points of information. The points of information are displayed within the matrix of the computer monitor. The image matrix consists of a number of pixels within the field of view (FOV). The FOV is the size of area which will display the pixels. The technologist controls the matrix size, FOV, and therefore, the pixel size of each image. The voxel is the volume element or third dimension of the matrix. The slice thickness alters the voxel size. Increasing the slice thickness will increase the voxel, whereas decreasing the slice thickness will decrease the voxel size. Therefore, anything that affects the slice thickness, matrix size, or the number of pixels within the matrix will affect the spatial resolution of the resulting image.

The technologist should remember that selection of any one of the scan parameters will affect image quality, scan time, and quantity of examinations performed. One of the major goals of diagnostic MRI is to acquire an image with the highest SNR, CNR, and highest possible spatial and contrast resolution in the shortest amount of time. In reality, there is a constant trade-off between these parameters to create the ideal image.

SELECTION OF THE OPTIMAL IMAGING COIL

There are numerous imaging coils available for the MR technologist to use for optimal imaging quality. There are coils that transmit and coils that transmit the RF pulse and receive the generated signal. Coils that function as transmitters and receivers are termed "transceivers." Common imaging coils include volume coils, surface coils, and phased array coils. Volume coils such as the head and body coils transmit the radio frequency pulse (RF) to a large area of anatomy at one given time. A large coil will cover a large area of interest; however, there is a trade-off associated with SNR and resolution. The SNR of a large coil has been improved with the use of a quadrature coil design. Patient positioning within the larger coil is not as critical as that of the smaller coil. This design uses the process of transmission and receiving by two different coils.

Surface coils are commonly used when imaging structures close to the surface of the patient. Imaging of extremities and spine work will often use surface coils. Because the coil is close to the area of interest, there is a significant improvement of SNR. Surface coils can be designed as rigid or flexible coils. Centering of the area of interest is important on extremity imaging when using smaller surface coils.

Phased array coils use multiple coils that combine and manipulate the information received from each coil to form one image. They can be linked together to increase the coverage of imaging and used in imaging of the spine or pelvis. The proper coil is determined by the anatomy being imaged and the patient's capabilities to physically complete the examination. The ideal coil for any MRI examination is one that will match the area of interest and efficiently receive the MR signal.

Proper safety measures should be included when working with imaging coils. When current passes through a loop of wire, the current will create its own magnetic field and RF field. Allowing the wire to form a loop or "coil" increases the risk of localized heating to the loop. The looped wire can result in patient burns caused by the thermal effects between the wire and patient's skin. This same principle applies to cables used to monitor the patient's vital signs during the MR examination. When using imaging coils, it is recommended to place a sheet or towel between the patient and the cable of the imaging coil. It is also recommended for the technologist to place padding between any area of the patient that may make contact with the bore of the magnet during image acquisition. The cable end of the coil should be laid out alongside of the patient if possible and not allowed to form a loop. The cable should be connected to the correct port and removed once the examination is completed.

CHAPTER 17

Patient Care Preparations

Patient care is a process that starts before and after the patient has left the imaging facility. This section focuses on the actual time frame the patient is present within the imaging facility. Because cardiopulmonary resuscitation is also a vital part of patient care, it is necessary for the technologist to be currently certified in cardiopulmonary resuscitation.

IDENTIFICATION OF THE PATIENT AND EVALUATION OF REQUISITION, MEDICAL RECORD, OR BOTH

The technologist actually starts the examination process before the patient physically arrives at the imaging center. Important information concerning the patient's medical needs and reason for the examination are routinely provided during the scheduling process. The patient's height, weight, and other pertinent information should also be collected at this time. This process allows the technologist the opportunity to compile a history on the patient. Before the examination, the technologist will locate available previous diagnostic examinations. Previous examinations are valuable for the radiologist and technologist to use as a comparative resource with current information. Information gathered before the MR examination can correlate the symptoms of the patient with the optimal examination. If there is any doubt concerning the requested examination or questions on medical history, the technologist should contact the referring physician and radiologist before examination of the patient.

SAFETY SCREENING AND PATIENT EDUCATION CONCERNING THE PROCEDURE

The following screening processes are oriented toward the patient, but it should be stressed that anyone accompanying the patient into the examination room is also subject to the same screening questions. The importance of patient screening is a process that cannot be stressed

FIGURE 17-1

MRI Procedure Screening Form

THE FOLLOWING ITEMS MAY BE HAZARDOUS OR MAY INTERFERE WITH THE MRI EXAMINATION BY PRODUCING AN ARTIFACT.

PLEASE INDICATE IF YOU HAVE ANY OF THE FOLLOWING:

YES   NO

_____   _____   Are you claustrophobic
_____   _____   Cardiac pacemaker
_____   _____   Aneurysm clips (Any head surgery)
_____   _____   Implanted cardiac defibrillator
_____   _____   Neurostimulator
_____   _____   Any type of biostimulator: _____
_____   _____   Any back or neck surgery

Any type of internal electrodes, including:

_____   _____   Pacing wires
_____   _____   Cochlear implants
_____   _____   Others _____
_____   _____   Implanted insulin pump
_____   _____   Swan-Ganz catheter
_____   _____   Any type of electronic, mechanical, or magnetic implant   Type:_____
_____   _____   Any type of intravascular coil, filter, or stent   Type: _____
_____   _____   Implanted drug infusion device
_____   _____   Any type of foreign body, shrapnel, or bullet
_____   _____   Heart valve prosthesis or heart surgery
_____   _____   Any type of ear implant
_____   _____   Penile prosthesis
_____   _____   Orbit/eye prosthesis
_____   _____   Any type of implant held in place by a magnet
_____   _____   Any type of surgical clip or staple
_____   _____   Vascular access port
_____   _____   Intraventricular shunt
_____   _____   Artificial limb or joint
_____   _____   Dentures
_____   _____   Diaphragm/IUD
_____   _____   Pessary
_____   _____   Wire mesh
_____   _____   Any implanted orthopedic items (i.e., pins, screws, nails, etc.)   Type:_____
_____   _____   Any other implanted item   Type: _____
_____   _____   Tattooed eyeliner (a small percentage of patients with tattooed eyeliner have experienced transient skin irritation in association with MRI. Therefore, you must decide if this slight risk warrants undergoing your examination. You may want to discuss this matter with your referring physician.)
_____   _____   Do you have a history of cancer (if yes, what was your primary site?_____)

Please complete questions on back and sign completed form.

YES   NO

Have you ever been injured by any metallic foreign body?   _____   _____
        (e.g., bullet, BB, shrapnel, etc.)
        Please describe:_____

Have you ever had an injury to the eye involving a metallic object   _____   _____
        (e.g., metallic slivers, shavings, foreign body, etc.)?
        Please describe:_____

Do you have anemia or diseases that affect your blood?   _____   _____

Do you have a history of renal disease, seizure, asthma, or respiratory disease?   _____   _____

Do you have any drug allergies?   _____   _____
        If yes, please list:_____

Have you ever had a reaction to a contrast medium used for MRI?   _____   _____

Are you pregnant or do you suspect you are pregnant?   _____   _____

Are you breast feeding?   _____   _____

We STRONGLY recommend using the ear plugs we supply for your MRI examination since some patients may find the noise levels unacceptable.

I attest the above information is correct to the best of my knowledge. I have read and understand the entire contents of this form and I have had the opportunity to ask questions regarding the information on this form.

Patient's Signature _____   Account Number _____

Witness _____

Weight:_____ lbs.

enough. Patient screening should occur multiple times before actually imaging the patient. Normally, the first set of screening questions is asked by the referring physician. The patient should again be screened when making the appointment for the MRI examination. Patients should be instructed to arrive at the imaging facility with a minimal amount of ferromagnetic items. They are normally instructed to be free of cosmetics, because some cosmetics will react to the RF pulse through the process of heat absorption. When the patient arrives at the imaging center, the screening process should be completed for the final time, before the patient is allowed to enter the MRI examination room. MR facilities have screening protocols in place to secure the safety of the patient and technologist from ferromagnetic items that may be brought in contact with the magnetic fringe field. Items for screening questions (Fig. 17-1) should include but not be limited to the following:

Identification of cardiac pacemakers

Presence of any electrically, magnetically, or mechanically activated implants

The presence of any implanted ferromagnetic materials that may torque, dislodge, or heat during the transmission of the RF pulse or the presence of the strong magnetic field

Screening precautions include the presence of any electrically, magnetically, or mechanically activated implants in any person intending to be in the proximity of the MR unit. The risk of malfunction of the implant is increased with influences of the static magnetic field. MRI is currently a contraindication for any person with a cardiac pacemaker.

All imaging facilities have a list of current contraindications to MR imaging. The technologist should be familiar with the book containing current contraindications of MR. Items such as cardiac pacemakers, cochlear implants, and aneurysm clips are contraindications for MR scanning. Ferromagnetic items that have become embedded in the patient, such as metal slivers may torque and heat. If there is a question of location within the patient, an x-ray examination or an alternative to an MRI examination may be necessary. Currently, it is not a contraindication for a pregnant patient to receive an MR examination. However, it is recommended the examination be postponed until after the first trimester or alternative imaging procedures such as ultrasound be used.

Before examination, request that the patient remove all personal items that may be ferromagnetic. Having the patient change into an examination gown is no clear assurance that all magnetic objects have been removed. A thorough visual "reinspection" is necessary before allowing the patient or anyone accompanying the patient to enter the examination room. The technologist should remember the magnet of the MR unit is not forgiving and seldom permits a second chance.

DOCUMENTATION OF PATIENT HISTORY, INCLUDING ALLERGIES

Attaining the patient history allows the technologist the opportunity to directly communicate with the patient. This process should be complete and not rushed. Many facilities use a form with questions referring to symptoms, combined with an anatomic drawing to allow the technologist and patient to mark and describe the areas of interest. Information on the history sheet should be direct and, most importantly, thorough. Questions concerning history of discomfort, previous surgeries, medications, and allergies should be included. Patient history concerning medications and allergies is useful in the process of patient monitoring, assessment, and for the use of contrast media or sedation for the examination. The questionnaire will allow the patient to participate and the opportunity to increase his or her level of confidence in the examination process.

The process of successful communication is apparent when involving the "claustrophobia question." Care must be taken to avoid the use of improper terminology when referring to the magnet within the MR unit. Often a poor choice of words can trigger a negative response from the patient. Questions concerning claustrophobia are an issue that should be determined by the individual imaging facility. Some facilities refrain from asking questions concerning claustrophobia unless the patient will be commuting from a substantial distance to the imaging center.

PATIENT ASSESSMENT

Claustrophobia affects between 5 and 10% of the patients having an MRI examination. Anxiety is a common physiologic effect of claustrophobia. Anxiety can make it difficult for the patient to remain motionless during the actual imaging process. The technologist should provide a complete description of the imaging unit along with an estimated length of examination. The patient should be informed about times between acquisitions and normal gradient noises. The use of hearing protection and mirrors can reduce the negative effects concerning claustrophobia. Reassure the patient they will be visually and verbally monitored. Maintaining the patient's confidence is an important part for the successful completion of the examination. Between acquisitions, the technologist should communicate with the patient regarding the progression of the examination. This communication allows the patient an opportunity for participation in the examination.

PATIENT POSITIONING

Patient positioning is dependent on the imaging procedure, the technologist, and the patient's capabilities. Manufacturers will provide guidelines for the ideal positioning for their specific equipment. It should always be considered a guideline. In the event the patient is unable to maintain a prone position, the technologist has the option to alter the position or not complete the examination. Rarely the latter is the only option. For example, when scanning the wrist, the patient has the option of placing the affected wrist along the side or overhead. Normal imaging of the head; neck; cervical, thoracic, or a combination of the whole spine; shoulders; chest; or abdomen is completed with the patient placed head first in the MR unit. Imaging of the lower extremities or lumbar spine is completed with the patient entering the MR unit feet first. The chapters containing the imaging procedures are based on a blend of technologist, radiologist, and manufacturer's recommendations. None of the procedures are set in stone, and they will constantly be adjusted to serve the needs of the patient, technologist, and radiologist. The procedures in the following chapters are to be used strictly as guidelines.

In addition to physically positioning the patient according to the examination protocol, it is wise to make sure the patient is comfortable before acquiring images. This is achieved by using any combination of positioning sponges, blankets, and restraining devices. The time it takes to make the patient comfortable will be returned through patient cooperation and reduction of patient movement.

DOCUMENTATION OF PROCEDURE: PATIENT DATA IN APPROPRIATE RECORDS

During the actual examination, it is important to complete the proper documentation of the examination process. MR facilities keep a log book for storing the statistical information of the specific examination. Information should include patient name, contrast, and scan information.

DISCHARGE THE PATIENT AND INFORM THE PATIENT OF ANY POSTPROCEDURAL INSTRUCTIONS

After the successful completion of the MR examination, removal of all positioning sponges and restraining devices is necessary. The patient should be allowed a moment to reorient him or herself to the setting before leaving the examination table. The technologist should inform the patient of the approximate time expected to obtain the results of the examination and any possible side effects from sedation or contrast injections.

UNIVERSAL PRECAUTIONS

When working with patients, the use of universal precautions is always important. These precautions are designed to protect health care workers from bloodborne pathogens. It is common practice to use universal precautions consistently for every patient with whom the technologist is in contact. There should be standard use of gloves when in contact with blood, bodily fluids, or nonintact skin. The use of gowns and protective eyewear may be necessary to complete a procedure that may involve blood or bodily fluids. Gowns should be removed after saturation or completion of examination. Needles should be properly disposed of at completion of use. After the completion of the examination, technologists should wash their hands. Each imaging facility should have a complete list of universal precautions to use as a reference before examination of patients.

CHAPTER 18

Examination Imaging Category

The image itself must be evaluated daily, this is done with the help of MR phantoms. The quality tests should be completed consistently, usually as part of the morning routine for the technologist. Results of the quality test should be stored for the required time and act as a reference to subtle changes within the image quality. In addition to routine quality testing, the technologist visually should inspect the quality of each image produced during the MR examination.

IMAGE DISPLAY, FILMING, AND ARCHIVING

The optimal study will include the appropriate imaging planes and image weighting as preferred by the imaging center. This means each image will display the appropriate field of view, proper slice thicknesses, and the images will be free of motion and have the proper annotation on each film. Upon completion of the examination, the technologist should record the images to the preferred filming format. Recording includes an image of the scan information menu and images in the preferred sequence. The technologist should inspect the developed films for appropriate quality. After successful filming of the study, the technologist should save the examination information on the proper data storage system. The data are stored for the length of time required by the imaging facility.

OPTIMAL IMAGE QUALITY, INCLUDING DEMONSTRATION OF ANATOMIC REGION

The quality of the examination is dependent on the diagnostic value of the images created. The optimal study will contain a combination of the best possible signal to noise ratio (SNR), contrast to noise ratio (CNR), and spatial resolution which could be completed in a reasonable amount of time. The resulting image should display the appropriate anatomy with the proper image weighting applied. The technologist should be aware the idealistic belief of attaining the optimal level of each parameter is not possible. Therefore, the technologist must determine which areas need to be optimal and levels of acceptability. Normally, the quality of the image will supersede the importance of speed. The quality of an image should be reproducible and consistent throughout a variety of examinations and patients.

PROPER IDENTIFICATION AND PATIENT DATA ON IMAGES

Each image should have the proper patient identification present. The information must be correct and current for the patient. Proper use of patient and facility data should also be consistent on each sheet of images. Additional patient data and scan information should be displayed according to radiologist preference and standards associated with the imaging center. Some imaging centers routinely place an abbreviated version of patient history and scan data on each image.

EXAMINATION COMPLETENESS

Upon the successful completion of the examination process, and after the dismissal of the patient, the technologist should prepare the MR room for the next examination. The examination room should have the bedding replaced, imaging coils stored in the proper location, and any contrast or injection materials should be removed and disposed of in the proper location. The past films, current films, and current patient history are collected and ready for the radiologist to view the study. The technologist is now ready for the next patient.

MR IMAGING PROCEDURES

The following procedures are recommended by the American Registry of Radiologic Technologists (ARRT) as the minimal requirements that the magnetic resonance technologist should be proficient at before the application of the advanced registry in magnetic resonance imaging. The intention of this manual is to meet the needs of the technologist and the ARRT. It is not the author's intention to dictate the preferences of the specific imaging center. Therefore, the procedural manual does not include the pulse sequences and other imaging parameters that are normally a collaborative effort between the radiologist and imaging technologist. The imaging planes that have been chosen are the most commonly used, which were selected from the technologist's preferences as well as those selected through research.

CHAPTER 19

MR Imaging Procedures of the Head and Neck

HEAD/ADULT

Mandatory minimum required is 10.

Common Indications

- Demonstration of gray matter, white matter, nerve tissue, basal ganglia, ventricles, and brainstem
- Unexplained neurologic symptoms, evaluation of infarction, AIDS (toxoplasmosis)
- Multiple sclerosis, primary tumor assessment, and metastatic disease

Imaging Considerations

The use of a standard head coil, centered to the main magnet, is recommended for brain imaging. Placement of saturation pulses inferior to the field of view (FOV) will also minimize flow artifacts from arteries. Adjust appropriate FOV setting for patient size (infant vs. adult), with consideration of signal to noise ratio (SNR). Image weighting protocols can be customized to demonstrate the area of interest with consideration of scan time. Paramagnetic contrast medium is used per facility requirements. An accurate explanation of the examination process, with consideration of patient comfort, will reduce voluntary motion during the imaging process.

Patient Preparations

The patient is placed supine and head first on the examination table with the head placed within the coil. The head is positioned with the midsagittal plane parallel with the longitudinal positioning lights. The interpupillary line is parallel with the horizontal positioning lights. Positioning pads and restraining straps should be used as needed. The patient's arms should be placed across the abdomen or at the sides of the patient. To minimize flow artifacts, the use of peripheral gating or saturation pulses may be considered.

Imaging Protocols

The localizer image should include the foramen magnum and the superior border of the parietal bones. Coronal and axial images are determined by the sagittal localizer image.

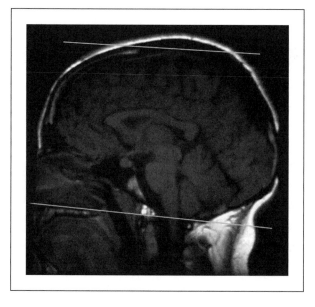

FIGURE 19-1

Sagittal image of head with appropriate range of slices from foramen magnum to superior portion of the brain tissue.

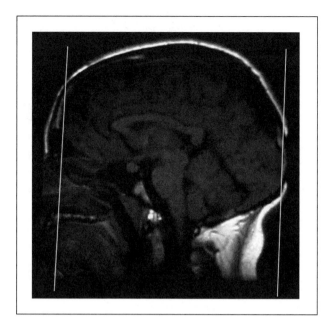

FIGURE 19-2

For MR Brain: sagittal image of head with range of slices extending from the anterior frontal lobe to the posterior portion of the cerebellum.

AXIAL/OBLIQUE IMAGES

A sagittal localizer image is used to determine the range of slices angled parallel with a line extending from the anterior to posterior commissure. Axial images are acquired from the foramen magnum to superior portion of the brain tissue (Fig. 19-1).

CORONAL IMAGES

A sagittal localizer image is used to determine the range of slices extending from the anterior frontal lobe to the posterior portion of the cerebellum (Fig. 19-2).

HEAD/CRANIAL NERVES

Elective minimum required is 4.

Common Indications

- Visualization of cranial nerves VII (facial) and VIII (auditory)
- Diagnosis of a posterior fossa lesion
- Trigeminal neuralgia
- Vertigo
- Unilateral sensory hearing loss
- Facial palsy

223

Imaging Considerations

The use of a standard head coil, centered to the main magnet, is recommended for imaging of the cranial nerves. The use of saturation pulses superior and inferior to the area of the internal auditory canal is recommended to minimize flow artifacts from CSF and blood. Use the appropriate FOV to maximize spatial resolution, with consideration of signal to noise ratio (SNR). Image weighting protocols can be customized to demonstrate the area of interest with consideration of scan time. Paramagnetic contrast medium is used per facility requirements. An accurate explanation of the examination process, with consideration of patient comfort, will reduce voluntary motion during the imaging process.

Patient Preparations

The patient is positioned in a manner similar to that for a normal brain examination. The patient is placed supine and head first on the examination table with the head placed within the coil. The head is positioned with midsagittal plane parallel with the longitudinal positioning lights. The interpupillary line is parallel with the horizontal positioning lights. Positioning pads and restraining straps should be used as needed. The patient's arms should be placed across the abdomen or at the sides of the patient. To minimize flow artifacts, the use of peripheral gating or saturation pulses may be considered.

Imaging Protocols

The localizer image should include the foramen magnum and the superior aspect of the head. Coronal and axial images are determined by the sagittal localizer image.

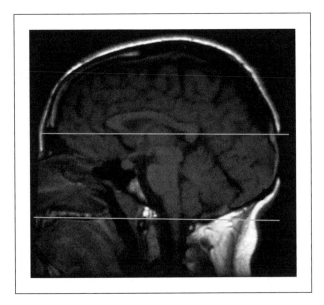

FIGURE 19-3

Sagittal image of head with appropriate range of slices extending from the foramen magnum through the petrous ridge.

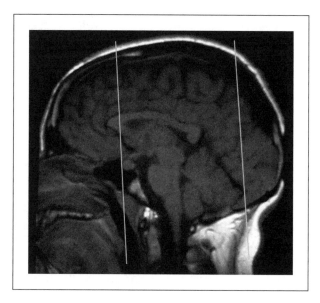

FIGURE 19-4

Sagittal image of head with appropriate range of slices extending from the clivus through the cerebellum.

AXIAL IMAGES

A sagittal localizer image is used to determine the range of thin slices extending from the foramen magnum through the petrous ridge (Fig. 19-3).

CORONAL IMAGES

A sagittal localizer image is used to determine the range of thin slices extending from the clivus through the cerebellum (Fig. 19-4).

HEAD/INTERNAL AUDITORY CANAL

Mandatory minimum required is 4.

Common Indications

- Visualization of cranial nerves VII (facial) and VIII (auditory)
- Diagnosis of a posterior fossa lesion
- Trigeminal neuralgia
- Vertigo
- Unilateral sensory hearing loss
- Facial palsy

Imaging Considerations

The use of a standard head coil, centered to the main magnet, is recommended for imaging of the internal auditory canal. The use of saturation pulses superior and inferior to the area of the internal auditory canal is recommended to minimize flow artifacts from cerebrospinal fluid and blood. Use the appropriate FOV to maximize spatial resolution, with consideration of SNR. Image weighting protocols can be customized to demonstrate the area of interest with consideration of scan time. Paramagnetic contrast medium is used per facility requirements. An accurate explanation of the examination process, with consideration of patient comfort, will reduce voluntary motion during the imaging process.

Patient Preparations

The patient is positioned in a manner similar to that for a normal brain examination. The patient is placed supine and head first on the examination table with the head placed within the coil. The head is positioned with midsagittal plane parallel with the longitudinal positioning lights. The interpupillary line is parallel with the horizontal positioning lights. Positioning pads and restraining straps should be used as needed. The patient's arms should be placed across the abdomen or at the sides of the patient. To minimize flow artifacts, the use of peripheral gating or saturation pulses may be considered.

Imaging Protocols

The localizer image should include the foramen magnum and the superior aspect of the head. Axial images are determined by the sagittal localizer image.

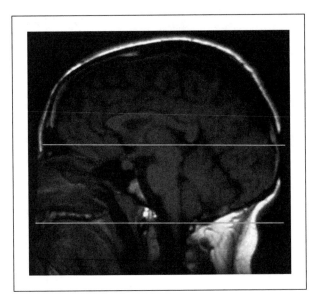

FIGURE 19-5

A sagittal image of head with appropriate range; slices extending from the foramen magnum through the petrous ridge.

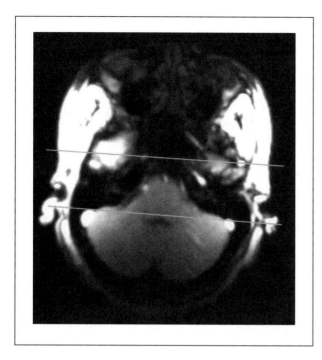

FIGURE 19-6

Axial image of head with appropriate range; slices extending from the clivus through the cerebellum.

AXIAL IMAGES

A sagittal localizer image is used to determine the range of thin slices extending from the foramen magnum through the petrous ridge (Fig. 19-5).

CORONAL IMAGES

An axial image is used to determine the range of thin slices extending from the clivus posteriorly through the external auditory meatus (Fig. 19-6).

HEAD/PITUITARY

Mandatory minimum required is 4.

Common Indications

- Visualization of optic nerve, infundibulum, pituitary gland, and clivus
- Diseases relating to pituitary function, hypothalamic disorders, and visual field defects.

Imaging Considerations

The use of a standard head coil, centered to the main magnet, is recommended for imaging of the pituitary gland. Placement of saturation pulses are recommended to minimize flow artifacts from blood. Because the pituitary is located anterior and inferior to the circle of Willis, the use of saturation pulses superior, inferior, left, and right of the pituitary are common. Use the appropriate FOV setting to maximize spatial resolution with consideration of SNR. Image weighting protocols can be customized to demonstrate the area of interest with consideration of scan time. Paramagnetic contrast medium is used per facility requirements. An accurate explanation of the examination process, with consideration of patient comfort, will reduce voluntary motion during the imaging process.

Patient Preparations

The patient is positioned in a manner similar to that for a normal brain examination. The patient is placed supine and head first on the examination table with the head placed within the coil. The head is positioned with midsagittal plane parallel with the longitudinal positioning lights. The interpupillary line is parallel with the horizontal positioning lights. Positioning pads and restraining straps should be used as needed. The patient's arms should be placed across the abdomen or at the sides of the patient. To minimize flow artifacts, the use of peripheral gating or saturation pulses may be considered.

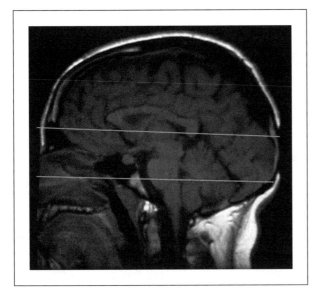

FIGURE 19-7

Sagittal image of head with appropriate range for axial slices extending from the floor of the pituitary fossa to the circle of Willis.

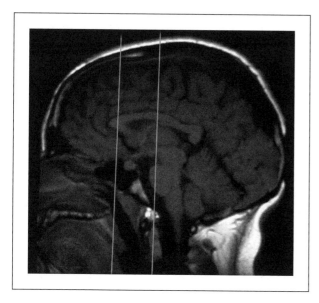

FIGURE 19-8

Sagittal image of head with appropriate range for coronal slices extending from the anterior to posterior clinoid processes.

The use of the smallest possible FOV to maximize spatial resolution with consideration to the number of excitations (NEX) is necessary to properly visualize the pituitary fossa. Most facilities use coronal and sagittal images to visualize the pituitary fossa. If axial images are required, images will extend from the floor of the pituitary fossa to the circle of Willis.

Imaging Protocols

The localizer image should include the foramen magnum and the superior border of the parietal bones. Coronal and axial images are determined by the sagittal localizer image.

AXIAL IMAGES

A sagittal localizer image is used to determine the range of thin slices extending from the floor of the pituitary fossa to the circle of Willis (Fig. 19-7).

CORONAL IMAGES

A sagittal localizer image is used to determine the range of thin slices extending from the anterior to posterior clinoid processes. The area extending from the inferior border of the sphenoid sinus to the superior border of the lateral ventricles should be included in the FOV (Fig. 19-8).

SAGITTAL IMAGES

A coronal image is used to determine the range of thin slices extending from the left to right lateral borders of the pituitary fossa. The

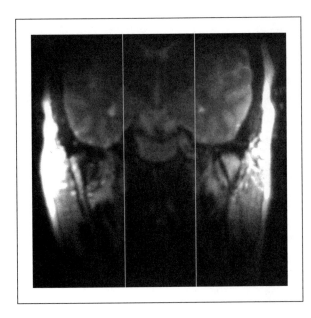

FIGURE 19-9

Coronal image of head with appropriate range for sagittal slices extending from the left to right lateral borders of the pituitary fossa.

area extending from the inferior border of the sphenoid sinus to the superior border of the lateral ventricle should be included in the FOV (Fig. 19-9).

HEAD/ORBIT

Mandatory minimum required is 4.

Common Indications

- Visualization of optic nerve
- Evaluation of orbital or ocular mass lesions
- Proptosis
- Visual disturbance

Imaging Considerations

The use of either a standard head coil, centered to the main magnet, or a surface coil placed over each orbit is an imaging option. Both eyes are examined for a comparison study of normal anatomy. To reduce motion, patients are instructed to assume a fixed-gaze position during signal acquisition.

Fat suppression is recommended to improve visualization of the optic nerve. The use of saturation pulses between the circle of Willis and posterior to the FOV are recommended to reduce artifacts in the area of the chiasm. In addition, inferior saturation pulses are recommended to minimize flow artifacts from blood and cerebrospinal fluid.

Use the appropriate FOV setting to maximize spatial resolution with consideration of SNR. Image weighting protocols can be customized to demonstrate the area of interest with consideration of scan time. Paramagnetic contrast medium is used per facility requirements. An accurate explanation of the examination process, with consideration of patient comfort, will reduce voluntary motion during the imaging process.

Patient Preparations

The patient is positioned in a manner similar to that for a normal brain examination. The patient is placed supine on the examination table with the head placed within the head coil. The head is positioned with midsagittal plane parallel with the longitudinal positioning lights. The horizontal positioning light should pass directly through the orbits or surface coil. Foam pads and restraining straps should be positioned as needed. The patient's arms should be placed across the abdomen or at the sides of the patient. To minimize flow artifacts, the use of peripheral gating or saturation pulses may be considered.

Imaging Protocols

The localizer image should include the foramen magnum and the superior border of the parietal bones. Coronal and axial or axial/oblique images are determined by the sagittal localizer image.

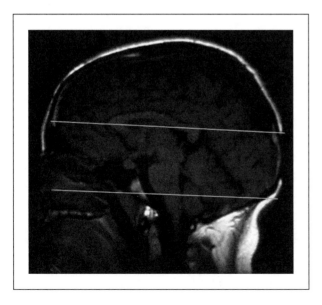

FIGURE 19-10

Sagittal image of head with appropriate range; slices extending from the inferior to superior orbital borders.

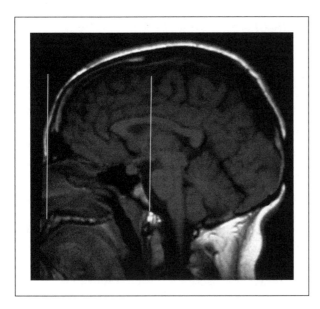

FIGURE 19-11

Sagittal image of head with appropriate range; coronal slices extending from the anterior border of the globe to the posterior aspect of the optic chiasm.

AXIAL/OBLIQUE IMAGES

A sagittal localizer image is used to determine the range of axial/oblique slices extending from the inferior to superior orbital borders. True axial or oblique slices are determined by medical protocols (Fig. 19-10).

CORONAL IMAGES

A sagittal localizer image is used to determine the range of coronal slices extending from the anterior border of the globe to the posterior aspect of the optic chiasm (Fig. 19-11).

SOFT TISSUE NECK

Elective minimum required is 3.

Common Indications

- Superior visualization of soft tissues of the neck, including muscles, vessels, and glands
- Staging of carcinoma of larynx
- Assessment of parapharyngeal masses, salivary gland masses, and neoplasms and nodal involvement

Imaging Considerations

The use of a standard neck coil, centered to the main magnet, is recommended for imaging of the neck. The appropriate FOV setting should be used to maximize spatial resolution with consideration of SNR. Image weighting protocols can be customized to demonstrate the area of interest within the neck with consideration of scan time. Paramagnetic contrast medium is used per facility requirements. An accurate explanation of the examination process, with consideration of patient comfort, will reduce voluntary motion during the imaging process.

Patient Preparations

The patient is placed supine and head first on the examination table. The neck is positioned with midsagittal plane parallel with the longitudinal positioning lights. The patient is positioned so the horizontal positioning light intersects the thyroid cartilage. The vertical positioning light should be midway between the anterior and posterior borders of the neck. Foam pads and restraining straps should be positioned as needed. The patient's arms should be placed across the abdomen or at the sides of the patient. To minimize flow artifacts, the use of peripheral gating or saturation pulses may be considered.

Imaging Protocols

The localizer image should include an area from the foramen magnum through the first thoracic vertebra. Coronal and axial images are determined by the sagittal localizer image.

AXIAL IMAGES

A sagittal localizer image is used to determine the range of axial slices extending from the inferior aspect of the first thoracic vertebra to the

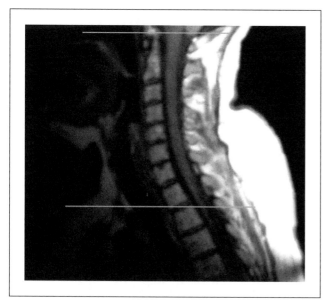

FIGURE 19-12

Sagittal image of neck from the foramen magnum through T1, with the appropriate range of axial slices extending from the inferior aspect of the first thoracic vertebra to the foramen magnum.

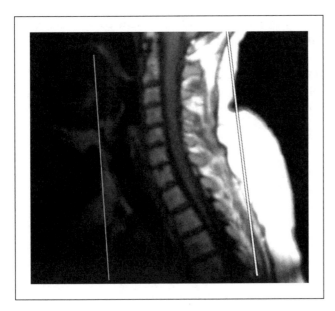

FIGURE 19-13

Sagittal image of neck from the foramen magnum through T1, with appropriate range; coronal slices extending from the anterior to posterior border of the neck.

foramen magnum. Flow compensation should be placed superior and inferior to the slice to minimize motion artifacts produced by carotid arteries and cerebrospinal fluid (Fig. 19-12).

CORONAL IMAGES

A sagittal localizer image is used to determine the range of coronal slices extending from the anterior to posterior border of the neck. Abnormalities can be localized with comparison of axial images (Fig. 19-13).

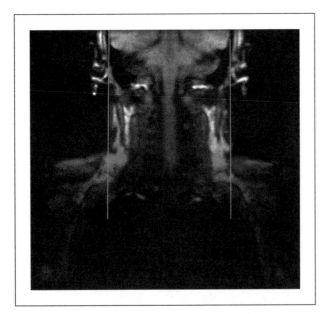

FIGURE 19-14

Coronal image of neck from the foramen magnum through T1, with appropriate range; sagittal slices extending from right to left lateral borders of neck.

SAGITTAL IMAGES

A coronal image is used to determine the range of slices extending from right to left lateral borders of neck. Sagittal images demonstrate side-to-side relationships of paraspinal soft tissues (Fig. 19-14).

VASCULAR IMAGING OF THE HEAD

Mandatory minimum required is 4 between head and neck vascular imaging.

Common Indications

- Evaluation of intracranial vasculature
- Evaluate the basilar artery and carotid siphon
- Arteriovenous malformations
- Assessment of aneurysms and infarcts
- Easement of occlusions

Imaging Considerations

For evaluation of intracranial vasculature, the use of a standard head coil, centered to the main magnet, is preferred. The carotid arteries and intracranial vascular structures are frequently used on the same study. Image weighting protocols can be customized to demonstrate the area of interest with consideration of scan time. Paramagnetic contrast medium is used per facility requirements. An accurate explanation of the examination process, with consideration of patient comfort, will reduce voluntary motion during the imaging process.

Patient Preparations

The patient is positioned in a manner similar to that for a normal brain examination. The patient is placed supine and head first on the examination table, with the head placed within the head coil. The head is positioned with midsagittal plane parallel with the longitudinal positioning lights. The interpupillary line is parallel with the horizontal positioning lights. Foam pads and restraining straps should be positioned as needed. The patient's arms should be placed across the abdomen or along the sides of the patient. To minimize flow artifacts, the use of peripheral gating or saturation pulses may be considered.

Imaging Protocols

A sagittal localizer image is used to determine the range of axial source images, which are viewed from the transverse and sagittal planes. Most vascular imaging of the head will include the vascular imaging of the neck; therefore, most examinations require both time of flight and 3D phase contrast. Vascular flow will be encoded in all three axes with 3D phase contrast; therefore, 3D phase contrast is often the choice for volume imaging of the head. In addition, 3D phase contrast is more sensitive to slow flow such as a large aneurysm. Three-dimensional time of flight may be the choice of imaging for evaluating fast flow–related vasculature such as small aneurysms and partial occlusions. The use of 3D time of flight will allow improved SNR and contiguous thin slices; however, the likelihood of intraslab flow is increased. The use of 2D time of flight imaging will maximize the visualization of slow venous flow or peripheral vessels.

VASCULAR IMAGING OF THE NECK

Mandatory minimum required is 4.

Common Indications

- Evaluation of neck vasculature, especially the bifurcation of the carotid arteries
- Evaluate the basilar artery and carotid siphon
- Arteriovenous malformations
- Aneurysms
- Occlusions

Imaging Considerations

For evaluation of carotid arteries, the use of a designated neck or MRA coil should be considered. The carotid arteries and intracranial vascular structures are frequently used on the same study. Image weighting protocols can be customized to demonstrate the area of interest within the neck with consideration of scan time. Paramagnetic contrast medium is used per facility requirements. An accurate explanation of the examination process, with consideration of patient comfort, will reduce voluntary motion during the imaging process.

Patient Preparations

The patient is placed supine and head first on the examination table. The neck is positioned with the midsagittal plane parallel to the longitudinal positioning lights. The patient should be positioned so that the horizontal positioning light intersects the angle of the mandible. The vertical positioning light should be midway between the anterior and posterior borders of the neck. Foam pads and restraining straps should be positioned as needed. The patient's arms should be placed across the abdomen or at the sides of the patient. To minimize flow artifacts, the use of peripheral gating or saturation pulses may be considered.

Imaging Protocols

A sagittal localizer image is used to determine the range of axial source images, which are viewed from the transverse and sagittal planes. The localizer image should include the base of the skull to the aortic arch. Saturation pulses should be located superior to the FOV to minimize artifacts from venous flow entering the volume of information. Most vascular imaging of the neck will include the vascular imaging of the head; therefore, most examinations require both time of flight and 3D phase contrast. Vascular flow will be encoded in all three axes with 3D phase contrast; therefore, 3D phase contrast is often the choice for volume imaging of the head. In addition, 3D phase contrast is more sensitive to slow flow such as a large aneurysm. For evaluating fast flow–related vasculature such as small aneurysms and partial occlusions, 3D time of flight may be the choice of imaging. The use of 3D time of flight will allow improved SNR and contiguous thin slices; however, the likelihood of intraslab flow is increased. The use of 2D time of flight imaging will maximize the visualization of slow venous flow or peripheral vessels.

CHAPTER 20

MR Imaging Procedures of the Spine

CERVICAL SPINE

Mandatory minimum required is 10.

Common Indications

- Evaluation of vertebral disks, ligaments, nerve roots, and cervical cord compression
- Assessment of spinal infection
- Visualization of multiple sclerosis plaques within the spinal cord
- Trauma to spinal cord
- Diagnosis of Arnold-Chiari malformation

Imaging Considerations

For evaluation of the cervical spine, a dedicated neck coil should be used. These coils can include a posterior cervical neck coil, volume neck coil, or phased array spinal coil. The coil should extend from the base of the skull to the area of the second thoracic vertebra. Image weighting protocols can be customized to demonstrate the area of interest within the cervical area with consideration of scan time. Paramagnetic contrast medium is used per facility requirements. Use of contrast medium will differentiate recurrent disk disease from postsurgical scarring. Scar tissue will enhance, whereas the disk will not. In addition, contrast medium will enhance metastatic lesions and multiple sclerosis plaques. An accurate explanation of the examination process, with consideration of patient comfort, will reduce voluntary motion during the imaging process.

Patient Preparation

The patient is positioned supine, with the midsagittal plane of the cervical spine aligned parallel with the longitudinal positioning light. Padding placed posterior to the patient's shoulders will aid in flattening of the cervical spine toward the neck coil. The horizontal alignment light should pass through the level of the hyoid bone. Foam pads and restraining straps should be positioned as needed. The patient's arms should be placed across the abdomen or at sides of the patient. To minimize flow artifacts, the use of peripheral gating or saturation pulses may be considered. For axial images, a saturation pulse placed anterior to the cervical spine will reduce motion artifacts generated from swallowing. The use of a rectangular field of view (FOV) will allow for a finer matrix and reduced scan times.

Imaging Protocols

The localizer image is used to ensure all cervical vertebral bodies have been included in the FOV. The image should include anatomy from the base of the skull through the first thoracic vertebra.

AXIAL/OBLIQUE IMAGES

A sagittal localizer image is used to determine the range of axial or axial/oblique images. For axial/oblique images, the range should be angled to produce images parallel with the intervertebral disk. Facilities often use three or four slices through the area of each vertebral disk or cord lesion (Fig. 20-1).

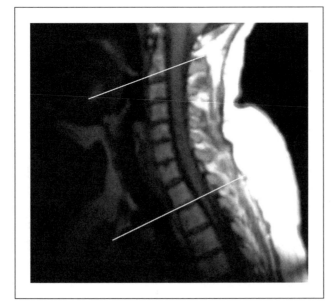

FIGURE 20-1

A sagittal localizer image is used to determine the range of axial or axial/oblique images. For axial/oblique images, the range should be angled to produce images parallel with the intervertebral disk. Facilities often use three or four slices through the area of each vertebral disk or cord lesion.

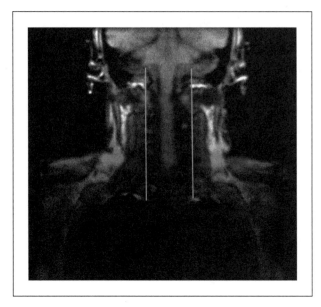

FIGURE 20-2

A coronal image will ensure that the cervical spine is positioned straight for future sagittal images. Images should be acquired from a range extending from the left lateral to right lateral borders of the vertebral bodies. Coronal image of cervical spine with appropriate range.

SAGITTAL IMAGES

A coronal localizer image will ensure that the cervical spine is positioned straight for future sagittal images. Images should be acquired from a range extending from the left lateral to the right lateral borders of the vertebral bodies. Use of a rectangular FOV will allow for a finer matrix and reduced scan times (Fig. 20-2).

THORACIC SPINE

Mandatory minimum required is 6.

Common Indications

- Evaluation of vertebral disks, ligaments, nerve roots, cord compression
- Assessment of spinal infection
- Visualization of multiple sclerosis plaques within the spinal cord

Imaging Considerations

For evaluation of the thoracic spine, use of a posterior spinal coil is recommended. The coil should extend from the superior aspect of the shoulders to the inferior costal angle. Image weighting protocols can be customized to demonstrate the area of interest within the thoracic area with consideration of scan time. Paramagnetic contrast medium is used per facility requirements. Use of contrast medium will differentiate recurrent disk disease from postsurgical scarring. The scar tissue will enhance, whereas the disk will not. In addition, contrast medium will enhance metastatic lesions and multiple sclerosis plaques. An accurate explanation of the examination process, with consideration of patient comfort, will reduce voluntary motion during the imaging process.

Patient Preparations

The patient is positioned supine with the head or feet first. The midsagittal plane of the spine is aligned parallel with the longitudinal positioning light. Padding placed posterior to the patient's shoulders will aid in flattening of the lower cervical and upper thoracic spine. The horizontal alignment light should pass through the level of the fourth thoracic vertebra or half-way between the sternal notch and xiphoid process. Foam pads and restraining straps should be positioned as needed. The patient's arms should be placed above the head. To minimize flow artifacts, the use of peripheral gating or saturation pulses may be considered.

Imaging Protocols

The localizer image is used to ensure that all thoracic vertebral bodies have been included in the FOV. It may be necessary to create a localizer extending from the base of the skull to determine the correct thoracic vertebra. A coronal localizer to ensure that the spine is positioned straight for future sagittal images.

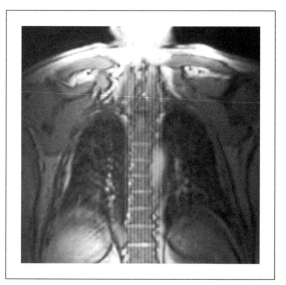

FIGURE 20-3

A coronal localizer image for sagittal images. Sagittal images should be acquired from a range extending from the left lateral to right lateral borders of the vertebral bodies.

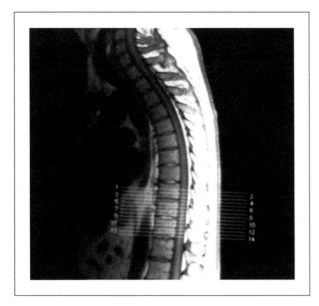

FIGURE 20-4

A sagittal localizer image is used to determine the range of axial or axial/oblique images. For axial/oblique images, the range should be angled to produce images parallel with the intervertebral disk. Facilities often use three or four slices through the area of each vertebral disk or cord lesion.

SAGITTAL IMAGES

A coronal localizer image will ensure that the spine is positioned straight for future sagittal images. Sagittal images should be acquired from a range extending from the left lateral to right lateral borders of the vertebral bodies. Use of a rectangular FOV will allow for a finer matrix and reduced scan times (Fig. 20-3).

AXIAL/OBLIQUE IMAGES

A sagittal localizer image is used to determine the range of axial or axial/oblique images. For axial/oblique images, the range should be angled to produce images parallel with the intervertebral disk. Facilities often use three or four slices through the area of each vertebral disk or cord lesion (Fig. 20-4).

LUMBOSACRAL SPINE

Mandatory minimum required is 10.

Common Indications

- Evaluation of conus, vertebral disks, ligaments, and nerve roots
- Cord compression
- Assessment of spinal infection

Imaging Considerations

For evaluation of the lumbosacral spine, the use of a thoracic/lumbar coil or complete spine coil is recommended. The coil should extend from a line posterior to the xiphoid tip through the inferior sacrum. Image weighting protocols can be customized to demonstrate the area of interest within the lumbosacral area with consideration of scan time. Paramagnetic contrast medium is used per facility requirements. Use of contrast medium will differentiate recurrent disk disease from postsurgical scarring. The scar tissue will enhance, whereas the disk will not. Contrast is also used to visualize lesions of the spinal cord. An accurate explanation of the examination process before the examination, as well as consideration of patient comfort, will reduce voluntary motion during the imaging process.

Patient Preparations

The patient is positioned supine and feet first, with the midsagittal plane of the spine aligned parallel with the longitudinal positioning light. The horizontal alignment light should pass through the level of the third lumbar vertebra. Padding placed posterior to the patient's knees will aid in flattening of the lumbar spine. Foam pads and restraining straps should be positioned as needed. The patient's arms should be placed across the upper abdomen or above the head of the patient. To minimize flow artifacts, the use of peripheral gating or saturation pulses may be considered. Use of rectangular FOV will allow for a finer matrix and reduced scan times.

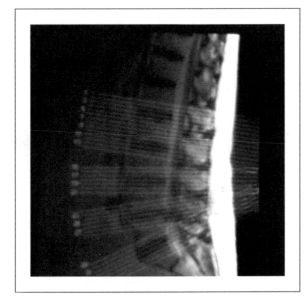

FIGURE 20-5

A sagittal localizer image is used to determine the range of axial or axial/oblique images. For axial/oblique images, the range should be angled to produce images parallel with the intervertebral disk. Facilities often use three or four slices through the vertebral disk or cord lesion. Images from only the lower three lumbar disks are normally examined.

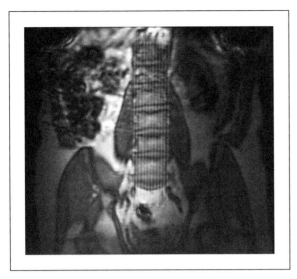

FIGURE 20-6

A coronal localizer image will ensure that the spine is positioned straight for future sagittal images. Sagittal images should be acquired from a range extending from the left lateral to right lateral borders of the vertebral bodies.

Imaging Protocols

A coronal localizer is used to ensure that the spine is positioned straight for future sagittal images. The localizer image should include an area from superior border of T12 and extend through the coccyx.

AXIAL/OBLIQUE IMAGES

A sagittal localizer image is used to determine the range of axial or axial/oblique images. For axial/oblique images, the range should be angled to produce images parallel with the intervertebral disk. Facilities often use three or four slices through the vertebral disk or cord lesion. Images from only the lower three lumbar disks are normally examined (Fig. 20-5).

SAGITTAL IMAGES

A coronal localizer image will ensure that the spine is positioned straight for future sagittal images. Sagittal images should be acquired from a range extending from the left lateral to the right lateral borders of the vertebral bodies (Fig. 20-6).

CHAPTER 21

MR Imaging Procedures of the Thorax

BRACHIAL PLEXUS

Elective minimum required is 3.

Common Indications

- Visualization of brachial plexus from the central origin, laterally toward the shoulders
- Diagnosis of brachial plexus lesions
- Evaluation of brachial plexus after trauma
- Thoracic outlet syndrome

Imaging Considerations

Visualization of the brachial plexus is best in the coronal plane. This is the main reason MRI is the examination of choice. Either the body coil, volume neck coil, or anterior neck coil can be used for examination of the brachial plexus. Image weighting protocols can be customized to demonstrate the area of interest with consideration of scan time. An accurate explanation of the examination process, with consideration of patient comfort, will reduce voluntary motion during the imaging process.

Patient Preparations

The patient is positioned supine and head first, with the midsagittal plane of the body aligned parallel with the longitudinal positioning light. The horizontal alignment light should pass through the sternal notch. Foam pads and restraining straps should be positioned as needed. The patient's arms should be placed along the sides of the patient. To minimize artifacts the use of respiratory compensation

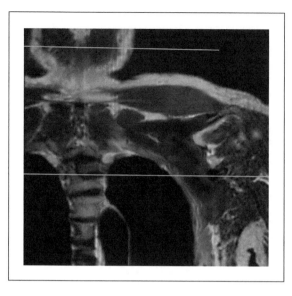

FIGURE 21-1

A coronal localizer image is used to determine the range of axial images. The axial images should extend from the third cervical vertebra through the sternoclavicular joints.

may be used. To minimize flow artifacts, the use of peripheral gating or saturation pulses should be considered.

Imaging Protocols

The localizer image should include an area from the third cervical vertebra through the sternoclavicular joints. Coronal and axial images are commonly used to evaluate the brachial plexus.

AXIAL IMAGES

A coronal localizer image is used to determine the range of axial images. Axial images are used for comparison of anatomic structures. The axial images should extend from the third cervical vertebra through the sternoclavicular joints (Fig. 21-1).

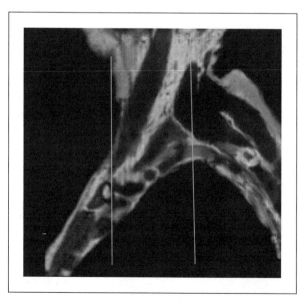

FIGURE 21-2

A sagittal image is used to determine the range of coronal images. Coronal images should extend from the sternoclavicular joints through the spinal cord.

CORONAL IMAGES

A sagittal image is used to determine the range of coronal images. Coronal images should extend from the sternoclavicular joints through the spinal cord (Fig. 21-2).

MEDIASTINUM

Elective minimum required is 3.

Common Indications

- Visualization of lymph nodes, great vessels, trachea, and thymus
- Detection of mediastinal lymphadenopathy
- Bronchial tumors
- Distinction between neoplasm and consolidated lung

Imaging Considerations

The use of the body coil along with respiratory compensation bellows and ECG/peripheral gating leads is recommended for examination of the mediastinum. Image weighting protocols can be customized to demonstrate the area of interest within the mediastinum with consideration of scan time. Paramagnetic contrast medium is used per facility requirements. Because the chest has a poor proton density, thicker slices should be considered to improve SNR. An accurate explanation of the examination process, with consideration of patient comfort, will reduce voluntary motion during the imaging process.

Patient Preparations

The patient is positioned supine and head first, with the midsagittal plane of the spine aligned parallel with the longitudinal positioning light. The horizontal alignment light should pass through the level of the fourth thoracic vertebra. Foam pads and restraining straps should be positioned as needed. The patient's arms should be placed along the sides of the patient. To minimize flow artifacts, the use of peripheral gating or saturation pulses may be considered.

Imaging Protocols

The localizer image should include an area from the superior border of the shoulders and extend through the apex of the diaphragm. Visualization of anatomy is common in both axial and coronal planes.

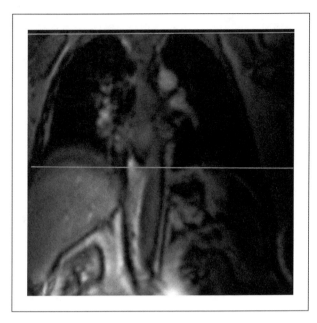

FIGURE 21-3

A coronal localizer image is used to determine the range of axial images. Axial images should be taken from a range extending from the apex of the lungs and ending at the diaphragm or through the area of interest.

AXIAL IMAGES

A coronal localizer image is used to determine the range of axial images. Axial images should be taken from a range extending from the apex of the lungs and ending at the diaphragm or through the area of interest (Fig. 21-3).

CORONAL IMAGES

An axial image is used to determine the range of coronal images. Coronal images extend from the range of the posterior chest muscles to the sternum (Fig. 21-4).

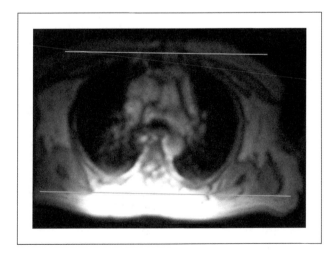

FIGURE 21-4

An axial image is used to determine the range of coronal images. Coronal images extend from the range of the posterior chest muscles to the sternum.

HEART

Elective minimum required is 3.

Common Indications

- Visualization of cardiac valves, papillary muscles and evaluation of myocardial blood supply from the right and left coronary arteries
- Diagnosis of arterial or ventricular septal defect
- Assessment of congenital abnormalities of the heart and great vessels

Imaging Considerations

The heart can be imaged by using the body coil, volume coil, or a spine coil. When using the spine coil, the patient should be placed in a prone position, thus placing the heart closer to the coil. Respiratory compensation bellows and ECG/peripheral gating leads are used per facility requirements. Image weighting protocols can be customized to demonstrate the area of interest with consideration of scan time. Paramagnetic contrast medium is used per facility requirements. An accurate explanation of the examination process, with consideration of patient comfort, will reduce voluntary motion during the imaging process.

Patient Preparations

Placement of ECG cables is done before imaging. The patient is seated on the examination table. Do *not* place the leads over the patient's ribs or scapula. The anterior placement of leads will provide an improved signal; however, motion from the chest must also be considered. The placement of respiratory bellows should be over the area of greatest breathing motion. The patient should now be placed supine and head first on the examination table with the mid-sagittal plane of the spine aligned parallel with the longitudinal positioning light. The horizontal alignment light should pass through the level of the xiphoid. Foam pads and restraining straps should be positioned as needed. The patient's arms should be placed along the sides of the patient. To minimize flow artifacts, the use of peripheral gating or saturation pulses may be considered.

Imaging Protocols

The localizer image should include the area from the shoulders through diaphragm. Because the heart lies in an oblique position, the optimal images are acquired in a single- or double-oblique orientation.

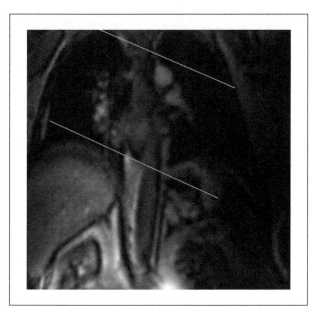

FIGURE 21-5

A coronal localizer image is used to determine the range of oblique images. Images should range parallel from the inferior border of the heart and extend through the aortic arch. Oblique images can be taken parallel and perpendicular to the interventricular septum. These images would range from the apex of the heart and extend through aortic arch.

Oblique imaging will produce true axial and longitudinal images of the heart.

The first image generated should be an axial image of the heart to visualize the ventricular septum. After this image the next two images are positioned obliquely. The first image (right anterior oblique view) is generated from a line parallel to the septum. The second image (left anterior oblique view) is generated from a line perpendicular to the septum.

OBLIQUE IMAGES

A coronal localizer image is used to determine the range of oblique images. Images should range parallel from the inferior border of the heart and extend through the aortic arch. Oblique images can be taken parallel and perpendicular to the interventricular septum. These images would range from the apex of the heart and extend through the aortic arch (Fig. 21-5).

VASCULAR IMAGING OF GREAT VESSELS

Elective minimum required is 3.

Common Indications

- Myocardial blood supply from the right and left coronary arteries
- Diagnosis of thoracic aortic aneurysm
- Evaluation of vessel patency and thrombus
- Assessment of congenital abnormalities of the heart and great vessels

Imaging Considerations

The great vessels can be imaged by using the body coil, volume coil, or a spine coil. When using the spine coil, the patient should be placed in a prone position, thus placing the heart closer to the coil. Respiratory compensation bellows and ECG/peripheral gating leads are used per facility requirements. Image weighting protocols can be customized to demonstrate the area of interest with consideration of scan time. Paramagnetic contrast medium is used per facility requirements. An accurate explanation of the examination process, with consideration of patient comfort, will reduce voluntary motion during the imaging process.

Patient Preparations

Placement of ECG cables is done before imaging. The patient is seated on the examination table. Do *not* place the leads over the patient's ribs or scapula. The anterior placement of leads will provide an improved signal; however, motion from the chest must also be considered. The placement of respiratory bellows should be over the area with the greatest breathing motion. The patient should now be placed supine and head first on the examination table, with the midsagittal plane of the spine aligned parallel with the longitudinal positioning light. The horizontal alignment light should pass through the level of the xiphoid. Foam pads and restraining straps should be positioned as needed. The patient's arms should be placed along the sides of the patient. To minimize flow artifacts, the use of peripheral gating or saturation pulses may be considered.

Imaging Protocols

The localizer image should include the area from the shoulders through the diaphragm. Because the heart lies in an oblique position, the optimal images are acquired in a single- or double-oblique orientation. Oblique imaging will produce true axial and longitudinal images of the heart and great vessels.

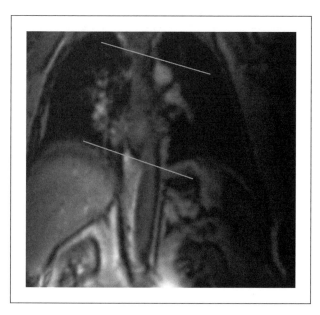

FIGURE 21-6

A coronal localizer image is used to determine the range of axial/oblique images. Oblique images extend from the border of the heart to the opposite border.

AXIAL/OBLIQUE IMAGES

A coronal localizer image is used to determine the range of axial/oblique images. Oblique images extend from the border of the heart to the opposite border (Fig. 21-6).

SAGITTAL/OBLIQUE IMAGES

An axial image taken through the ascending and descending aorta is used to determine the range of sagittal/oblique images of the aortic arch (Fig. 21-7).

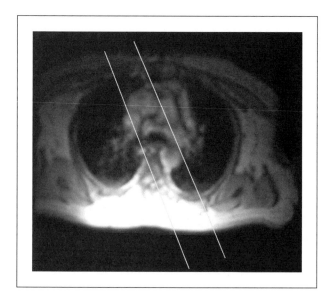

FIGURE 21-7

Axial image taken through the ascending and descending aorta is used to determine the range of sagittal/oblique images of the aortic arch.

BREAST

Elective minimum required is 3.

Common Indications

- Visualization and differentiation of glandular and adipose tissue
- Early detection of small lesions especially in patients whose breast tissue is too dense for adequate diagnosis through mammography
- Detection of leaks and rupture from silicon implants
- Alternative imaging procedure to mammography

Imaging Considerations

For imaging of the breast, the use of a designated breast coil, with the patient in a prone position and gown opening in the front is recommended. The technologist should place a rolled towel or pillow under the anterior surface of the patient's ankles to relieve pressure on legs and lower back. To reduce cervical pressure, position the patient so the head is lower than the rest of the body. For the detection of rupture or leaks from silicon implants, the technologist should consider the use of fat and water saturation pulses to distinguish escaping silicone from healthy breast tissue.

Image weighting protocols can be customized to demonstrate the area of interest with consideration of scan time. Paramagnetic contrast medium is used per facility requirements. An accurate explanation of the examination process, with consideration of patient comfort, will reduce voluntary motion during the imaging process.

Patient Preparations

The patient should be free of any deodorant, powder, or any breast jewelry during breast examination. The patient is positioned supine and head first on the examination table. The proper positioning of each breast is important before imaging. Breasts should be moved laterally and lifted superiorly to prevent pinching breast tissue between the chest wall and breast coil. The patient should support his or her head with crossed forearms, while at the same time keeping the body centered to the breast coil. The midsagittal plane of the spine is aligned parallel with the longitudinal positioning light. The horizontal alignment light should pass through the center of the breast coil. Foam pads and restraining straps should be positioned as needed.

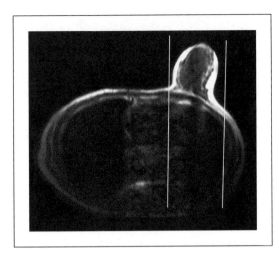

FIGURE 21-8

Axial image of the breast with an appropriate range; sagittal slices extending from lateral to medial borders of one or both breasts.

Imaging Protocols

The localizer image should include the entire area of breasts and axilla. Sagittal and axial images are normally used during breast imaging. The range of sagittal images can be determined from the axial localizer.

SAGITTAL IMAGES

The range for sagittal images of the breast can be determined from the axial localizer. The sagittal images should extend from the lateral to medial borders of one or both breasts. The images should include the axilla (Fig. 21-8).

AXIAL IMAGES

A sagittal image is used to determine the range of axial images. Axial images extend from the superior to inferior border of each or both breasts (Fig. 21-9).

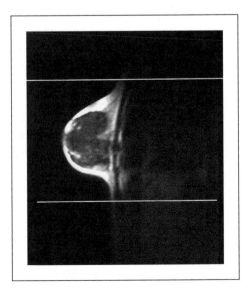

FIGURE 21-9

Sagittal image of the breast with an appropriate range; axial slices extending from superior to inferior borders of breasts.

CHAPTER 22

MR Imaging Procedures of the Abdomen

LIVER AND SPLEEN OR PANCREAS

Mandatory minimum required is 4.

Common Indications

- Visualization of organs within the abdominal cavity
- Assessment of focal lesions and staging of neoplasms
- Demonstration of liver metastasis

Imaging Considerations

Imaging of the liver and spleen is frequently completed with the body coil; however, the use of a dedicated torso coil can also be used. The patient is placed feet first and supine on examination table. The patient's arms can be raised above the head or along the sides of the patient. The torso coil should extend inferior from the midsternum. To reduce motion from breathing, the use of respiratory compensation bellows may be used. Image weighting protocols can be customized to demonstrate the area of interest within the abdomen with consideration of scan time. Paramagnetic contrast medium is used per facility requirements. An accurate explanation of the examination process, with consideration of patient comfort, will reduce voluntary motion during the imaging process.

Patient Preparations

The patient is positioned with the midsagittal plane aligned parallel with the longitudinal positioning light. Padding placed posterior to the patient's knees will reduce pressure in the area of the lumbar spine.

The horizontal alignment light should pass through the level of the third lumbar vertebra or lower costal margin. Foam pads and restraining straps should be positioned as needed. To minimize flow artifacts, the use of peripheral gating or saturation pulses may be considered.

Imaging Protocols

The coronal localizer image should include an area from mediastinum to symphysis pubis. The FOV should be adequate to include both lateral borders of the abdomen.

AXIAL IMAGES

A coronal localizer image is used to determine the range of axial images. The range of axial images should extend from the superior border of the diaphragm through the inferior aspect of the liver. The field of view (FOV) should be large enough to include the entire transverse image of the abdomen (Fig. 22-1).

CORONAL IMAGES

An axial image of the abdomen is used to determine the range of coronal images. Coronal images should extend from the posterior abdominal muscles to the anterior abdominal wall. The FOV is large enough on coronal images to include the superior border of the diaphragm and the symphysis at the inferior border (Fig. 22-2).

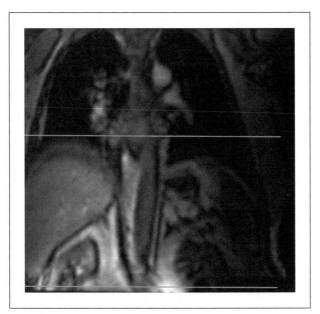

FIGURE 22-1

A coronal localizer image of the abdomen is used to determine the range of axial images. The range of axial images should extend from the superior border of the diaphragm through the inferior aspect of the liver. The FOV should be large enough to include the entire transverse image of the abdomen.

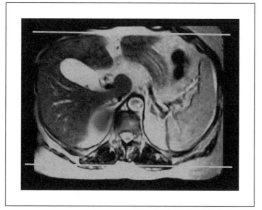

FIGURE 22-2

An axial image of the abdomen is used to determine the range of coronal images. Coronal images should extend from the posterior abdominal muscles to the anterior abdominal wall. The FOV is large enough on coronal images to include the superior border of the diaphragm and the symphysis at the inferior border.

KIDNEYS

Elective minimum required is 3.

Common Indications

- Assessment of renal masses as well as hemorrhage
- Staging and diagnosis of renal cell carcinoma

Imaging Considerations

Imaging of the kidneys is completed with a body coil, dedicated torso coil, or surface coil. If using the torso or surface coil, it should extend inferior from the midsternum. To reduce motion from breathing, the use of respiratory compensation bellows may be used. Image weighting protocols can be customized to demonstrate the area of interest within the abdomen with consideration of scan time. Paramagnetic contrast medium is used per facility requirements. An accurate explanation of the examination process, with consideration of patient comfort, will reduce voluntary motion during the imaging process.

Patient Preparations

The patient is placed feet first and supine on examination table. The patient's arms should be placed above the head of the patient. The patient is positioned with the midsagittal plane aligned parallel with the longitudinal positioning light. Padding placed posterior to the patient's knees will reduce pressure in the area of the lumbar spine. The horizontal alignment light should pass through the level of the third lumbar vertebra or lower costal margin. Foam pads and restraining straps should be positioned as needed. To minimize flow artifacts, the use of peripheral gating or saturation pulses may be considered.

Imaging Protocols

The coronal localizer image should include an area from the superior border of the diaphragm to the symphysis pubis. The FOV should be adequate to include both lateral borders of the abdomen.

AXIAL IMAGES

A coronal localizer image is used to determine the range of axial images. The range of axial images should extend from the superior aspect of the adrenal glands through the inferior border of the kidneys. The FOV is large enough to include the entire transverse image of the abdomen (Fig. 22-3).

CORONAL IMAGES

An axial image of the abdomen is used to determine the range of coronal images. Coronal images should extend from the posterior abdominal muscles to the anterior abdominal wall. The FOV is large enough on coronal images to include the superior border of the diaphragm and the symphysis at the inferior border (Fig. 22-4).

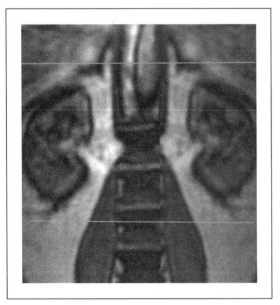

FIGURE 22-3

A coronal localizer image is used to determine the range of axial images. The range of axial images should extend from the superior aspect of the adrenal glands through the inferior border of the kidneys. The FOV is large enough to include the entire transverse image of the abdomen.

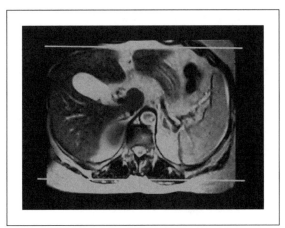

FIGURE 22-4

An axial image of the abdomen is used to determine the range of coronal images. Coronal images should extend from the posterior abdominal muscles to the anterior abdominal wall. The FOV is large enough on coronal images to include the superior border of the diaphragm and the symphysis at the inferior border.

ADRENAL GLANDS

Elective minimum required is 3.

Common Indications

- Demonstration of location of adrenal glands compared with the kidneys
- Assessment of renal and adrenal masses as well as hemorrhage

Imaging Considerations

Adrenal imaging is completed with a body coil, dedicated torso coil, or surface coil. The torso or surface coil should extend inferior from the midsternum. To reduce motion from breathing, the use of respiratory compensation bellows may be used. Image weighting protocols can be customized to demonstrate the area of interest within the abdomen with consideration of scan time. Paramagnetic contrast medium is used per facility requirements. An accurate explanation of the examination process, with consideration of patient comfort, will reduce voluntary motion during the imaging process.

Patient Preparations

The patient is placed feet first and supine on examination table. The patient's arms should be placed above the head of the patient. The patient is positioned with the midsagittal plane aligned parallel with the longitudinal positioning light. Padding placed posterior to the patient's knees will reduce pressure in the area of the lumbar spine.

The horizontal alignment light should pass through the level of the third lumbar vertebra or lower costal margin. Foam pads and restraining straps should be positioned as needed. To minimize flow artifacts, the use of peripheral gating or saturation pulses may be considered.

Imaging Protocols

The localizer image should include an area from the superior border of the diaphragm to symphysis pubis. The FOV should be adequate to include both lateral borders of the abdomen.

AXIAL IMAGES

A coronal localizer image is used to determine the range of axial images. The range of axial images should extend from the superior aspect of the adrenal glands through the inferior border of the kidneys. The FOV is large enough to include the entire transverse image of the abdomen (Fig. 22-5).

CORONAL IMAGES

An axial image through the kidneys is used to determine the range of coronal images. Coronal images should extend from the posterior abdominal muscles to the anterior abdominal wall. The FOV is large enough on coronal images to include the superior border of the diaphragm and the symphysis at the inferior border (Fig. 22-6).

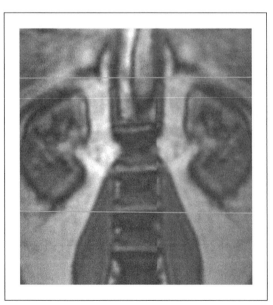

FIGURE 22-5

A coronal localizer image is used to determine the range of axial images. The range of axial images should extend from the superior aspect of the adrenal glands through the inferior border of the kidneys. The FOV is large enough to include the entire transverse image of the abdomen.

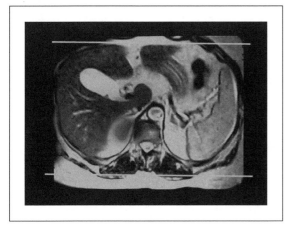

FIGURE 22-6

An axial image through the kidneys is used to determine the range of coronal images. Coronal images should extend from the posterior abdominal muscles to the anterior abdominal wall. The FOV is large enough on coronal images to include the superior border of the diaphragm and the symphysis at the inferior border.

VASCULAR IMAGING OF THE ABDOMEN AND PELVIS

Elective minimum required is 3.

Common Indications

- Assessment of vasculature such as the abdominal aorta, common iliac arteries, and femoral arteries
- Demonstration of major vascular anomalies
- Assessment of vasculature before transplant or resection
- Evaluation of abdominal aortic aneurysms

Imaging Considerations

Vascular imaging of the abdomen and pelvis is completed with a body coil, dedicated torso coil, dedicated pelvic coil, or surface coil. When using the torso or surface coil, it should extend inferior from the midsternum. To reduce motion from breathing, respiratory compensation bellows may be used. The pelvic coil should extend from the iliac crest through the symphysis. Image weighting protocols can be customized to demonstrate the area of interest within the abdomen and pelvis with consideration of scan time. Paramagnetic contrast medium is used per facility requirements. An accurate explanation of the examination process, with consideration of patient comfort, will reduce voluntary motion during the imaging process.

Patient Preparations

The patient is placed feet first and supine on examination table. The patient's arms should be placed above the head of the patient. The patient is positioned with the midsagittal plane aligned parallel with the longitudinal positioning light. Padding placed posterior to the patient's knees will reduce pressure in the area of the lumbar spine. The horizontal alignment light should pass through the level of the third lumbar vertebra or lower costal margin. Foam pads and restraining straps should be positioned as needed. To minimize flow artifacts, the use of saturation pulses may be considered.

Imaging Protocols

The localizer image should include the area from mediastinum to symphysis pubis. The FOV should be adequate to include both lateral borders of the abdomen.

AXIAL 2D OR 3D TIME OF FLIGHT MRA

A coronal localizer image is used to determine the range of axial images. The range of axial images should include the specific area of interest. The slices should be continuous or gathered in a volume of information at one given time. After gathering the information with the use of 2D or 3D time of flight MRA, it can be reconstructed into other desired imaging planes.

PELVIS

Mandatory minimum required is 4.

Common Indications

- Assessment of bladder wall and associated pathologic conditions
- Evaluation of urogenital tract, including diagnosis of carcinoma to the bladder, cervix, uterus, and rectum
- Localization of undescended testicles

Imaging Considerations

Pelvic imaging can be completed with the body coil or dedicated pelvic array coil. When using the pelvic coil, it should extend from the iliac crest through the symphysis. Image weighting protocols can be customized to demonstrate the area of interest within the pelvis with consideration of scan time. Paramagnetic contrast medium is used per facility requirements. An accurate explanation of the examination process, with consideration of patient comfort, will reduce voluntary motion during the imaging process.

Patient Preparations

The patient is placed feet first and supine on the examination table. The patient is positioned with the midsagittal plane aligned parallel with the longitudinal positioning light. Padding placed posterior to the patient's knees will reduce pressure in the area of the lumbar spine as well as flatten the pelvic area against the examination table. Horizontal alignment light should pass midway between the iliac crest and symphysis pubis. Foam pads and restraining straps should be positioned as needed. The patient's arms should be placed across the abdomen of the patient. To minimize flow artifacts, the use of peripheral gating or saturation pulses may be considered. Bowel motion can be reduced with compression or by instructing patient to concentrate on breathing from the chest and upper abdomen without pelvic movement.

Imaging Protocols

The coronal localizer image should include an area from umbilicus to inferior pelvic border. The FOV should be adequate to include both lateral borders of the abdomen. Axial and sagittal images are determined by the coronal localizer image.

AXIAL IMAGES

A coronal localizer image of the pelvis is used to determine the range of axial images. The range of axial images should extend from the iliac crest through the pelvic floor. The FOV is large enough to include the entire transverse image of the pelvis (Fig. 22-7).

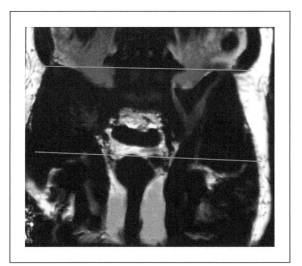

FIGURE 22-7

A coronal localizer image of the pelvis is used to determine the range of axial images. The range of axial images should extend from the iliac crest through the pelvic floor. The FOV is large enough to include the entire transverse image of the pelvis.

265

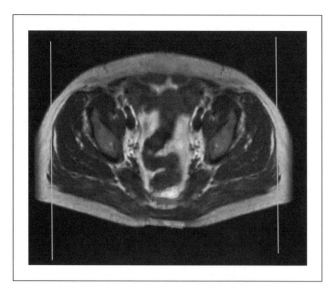

FIGURE 22-8

An axial image of the pelvis is used to determine the range of sagittal images. Sagittal images can be taken from lateral border to opposite lateral border of the pelvis or through the specific area of interest.

SAGITTAL IMAGES

An axial image of the pelvis is used to determine the range of sagittal images. Sagittal images can be taken from lateral border to opposite lateral border of the pelvis or through the specific area of interest. Sagittal images are useful in evaluation of midline structures such as uterus, cervix, and vagina (Fig. 22-8).

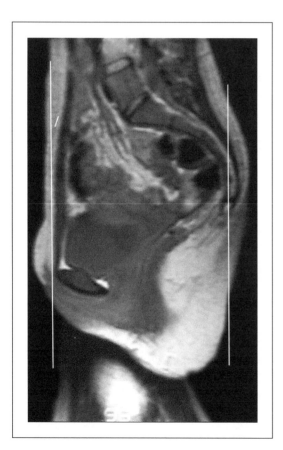

FIGURE 22-9

A sagittal image of the pelvis is used to determine the range of coronal images. Coronal images should extend from the anterior border of the symphysis pubis to the coccyx. The FOV should be large enough to include the iliac crest and symphysis pubis. Coronal images of the pelvis with a range of axial images should extend from the iliac crest through the pelvic floor.

CORONAL IMAGES

A sagittal image of the pelvis is used to determine the range of coronal images. Coronal images should extend from the anterior border of the symphysis pubis to the coccyx. The FOV should be large enough to include the iliac crest and symphysis pubis. Coronal images are used to evaluate the pelvic sidewall for invasion in cases of uterine or cervical carcinoma (Fig. 22-9).

PROSTATE

Elective minimum required is 3.

Common Indications

- Visualization of seminal vesicles, prostate, rectum, and base of the bladder
- Evaluation of capsular invasion and staging the results
- Evaluation of rectal fistulas

Imaging Considerations

Prostate imaging is completed with an endorectal coil or dedicated pelvic array coil. The pelvic coil should extend from the iliac crest through the symphysis. If the endorectal coil is to be used, it should be inserted carefully to avoid perforation of rectal tissue. Image weighting protocols can be customized to demonstrate the area of interest within the pelvis with consideration of scan time. Paramagnetic contrast medium is used per facility requirements. An accurate explanation of the examination process, with consideration of patient comfort, will reduce voluntary motion during the imaging process.

Patient Preparations

The patient is placed feet first and supine on examination table. The patient is positioned with the midsagittal plane aligned parallel with the longitudinal positioning light. Padding placed posterior to the patient's knees will reduce pressure in the area of the lumbar spine as well as flatten the pelvic area against the examination table. The horizontal alignment light should pass midway between the iliac crest and symphysis pubis. Foam pads and restraining straps should be positioned as needed. The patient's arms should be placed above the abdomen of the patient. To minimize flow artifacts, the use of peripheral gating or saturation pulses may be considered. Bowel motion can be reduced with compression or by instructing the patient to concentrate on breathing from the chest and upper abdomen without pelvic movement.

Imaging Protocols

The sagittal localizer should include an area from umbilicus to inferior pelvic border. When using the endorectal coil, the localizer should include the posterior bladder wall to the posterior wall of the rectum.

AXIAL IMAGES

A sagittal localizer image of the pelvis is used to determine the range of axial images. The range of axial images should extend inferior from the superior border of the seminal vesicles. If using the pelvic coil, the FOV should be large enough to include the entire transverse image of the pelvis (Fig. 22-10).

SAGITTAL IMAGES

An axial image is used to determine the range of sagittal images. Sagittal images should extend through the area of interest, from lateral to lateral border of the bladder (Fig. 22-11).

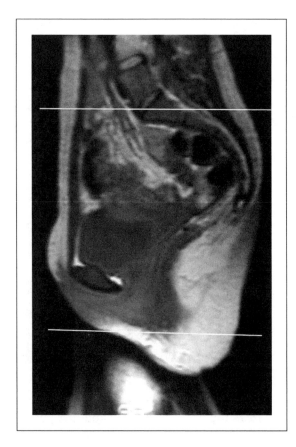

FIGURE 22-10

A sagittal localizer image of the pelvis is used to determine the range of axial images. The range of axial images should extend inferior from the superior border of the seminal vesicles. If using the pelvic coil, the FOV should be large enough to include the entire transverse image of the pelvis.

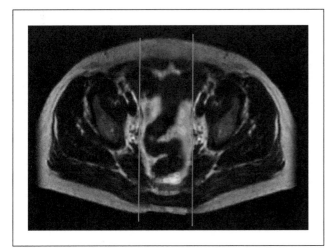

FIGURE 22-11

An axial image is used to determine the range of sagittal images. Sagittal images should extend through the area of interest, from lateral to lateral border of the bladder.

CORONAL IMAGES

A sagittal image of the pelvis is used to determine the range of images, which extend through the area of interest. This image should include the base of the bladder and its relationship to the prostate. Sagittal and coronal images are useful in evaluation of midline structures such as prostate, bladder, and rectum. Coronal images are also used to evaluate the pelvic sidewall (Fig. 22-12).

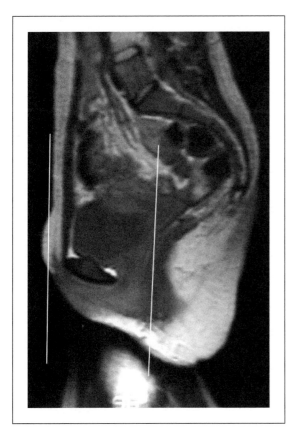

FIGURE 22-12

A sagittal image of the pelvis is used to determine the range of images, which extend through the area of interest. This should include the base of the bladder and its relationship to the prostate.

CHAPTER 23

MR Imaging Procedures of the Musculoskeletal System

TEMPOROMANDIBULAR JOINT

Elective minimum required is 3.

Common Indications

- Visualization of the articular tubercle, articular disk, and lateral pterygoid muscle
- Assessment of internal meniscal derangement

Imaging Considerations

Typically a temporomandibular joint (TMJ) study will include a complete head examination. Imaging is completed with dual 3-in. coils. The designated dual 3-in. coils should be placed parallel with the face of the coils as close to the surface of the patient without touching. Both joints should be centered to the coils and imaged simultaneously. Image weighting protocols can be customized to demonstrate the area of interest with consideration of scan time. Paramagnetic contrast medium is used per facility requirements. Instruct the patient to minimize swallowing during the imaging procedure. An accurate explanation of the examination process, with consideration of patient comfort, will reduce voluntary motion during the imaging process.

Patient Preparations

The patient is placed head first and supine on examination table. The patient's arms should lay across the abdomen or along the sides of the patient. Before imaging, instruct the patient of proper timing for opening and closing of the mouth. Use of a mouth-opening device may be necessary. The patient is positioned with the midsagittal plane aligned parallel with the longitudinal positioning light. Placing padding posterior to the patient's knees will reduce pressure in the area of the lumbar spine and improve patient comfort. The horizontal alignment light should pass through the level of the TMJs, centered within the coil. Foam pads and restraining straps should be positioned as needed. Use of saturation pulses and triggering is normally not necessary for TMJ imaging.

Imaging Protocols

The axial localizer image should include the entire area of the head from anterior and posterior borders.

SAGITTAL/OBLIQUE IMAGES

The axial localizer image is used to determine the range of sagittal/oblique images. The range of sagittal/oblique images should extend from the lateral to the medial border of the temporomandibular joint. Slices should be angled perpendicular to mandibular condyles. Both temporomandibular joints can be displayed on each image (Fig. 23-1).

CORONAL IMAGES

The axial localizer image can be used to determine the range of coronal images. Coronal images should be aligned parallel with the temporomandibular joint (Fig. 23-2).

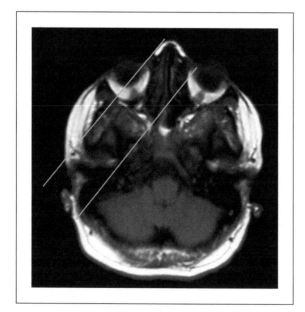

FIGURE 23-1

The axial localizer image is used to determine the range of sagittal/oblique images. The range of sagittal/oblique images should extend from the lateral to medial border of the temporomandibular joint. Slices should be angled perpendicular to mandibular condyles. Both temporomandibular joints can be displayed on each image.

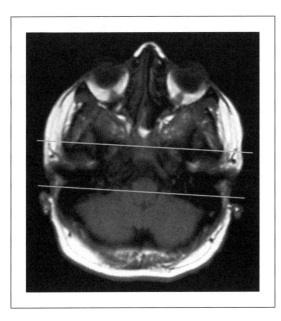

FIGURE 23-2

The axial image can be used to determine the range of coronal images. Coronal images should be aligned parallel with the temporomandibular joint.

SHOULDER

Mandatory minimum required is 6.

Common Indications

- Visualization of tendons, muscles, and cartilage
- Evaluation of impingement and shoulder instability

Imaging Considerations

Shoulder imaging is completed with either a dedicated shoulder coil, round surface, or flexible coil. Attach the proper coil before positioning the patient in the supine position. The shoulder coil is centered over the affected humeral head. Image weighting protocols can be customized to demonstrate the area of interest with consideration of scan time. Paramagnetic contrast medium should be used per facility requirements. An accurate explanation of the examination process, with consideration of patient comfort, will reduce voluntary motion during the imaging process.

Patient Preparations

The patient is positioned supine head first into the magnet. Align the patient so that the affected shoulder is as close to the magnetic isocenter as possible. Measurement of the offset distance should be compensated for before imaging. The longitudinal alignment light should lie midline to the patient's body and not the shoulder. The horizontal alignment light should pass through the shoulder joint. Placing padding posterior to the patient's humerus and elbow will support and reduce motion by adding to patient comfort. To minimize flow artifacts, the use of saturation pulses may be considered. The use of respiratory compensation is another option for reducing motion.

Imaging Protocols

The axial localizer image should include the acromion to the humeral neck.

CORONAL/OBLIQUE IMAGES

An axial localizer image is used to determine the range of coronal/oblique images. Coronal/oblique images should be parallel to the supraspinatus muscle and extend from posterior to anterior borders of the joint or through the area of interest. Oblique the plane as needed, while placing the joint space in the center of the field of view (Fig. 23-3).

SAGITTAL/OBLIQUE IMAGES

The axial localizer image is used to determine the range of sagittal/oblique images. Sagittal/oblique images should be parallel with the joint space and extend medially from the glenoid cavity laterally to the bicipital groove (Fig. 23-4).

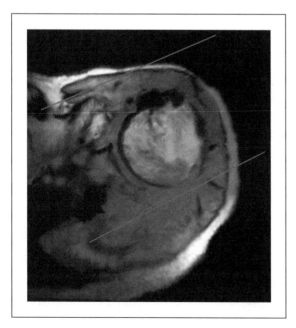

FIGURE 23-3

An axial localizer image is used to determine the range of coronal/oblique images. Coronal/oblique images should be parallel to the supraspinatus muscle and extend from the posterior to anterior borders of the joint or through the area of interest. Oblique the plane as needed, while placing the FOV center at the joint space.

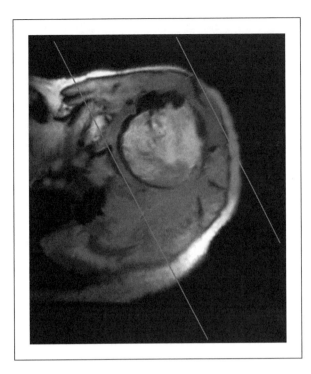

FIGURE 23-4

An axial localizer image is used to determine the range of sagittal/oblique images. Sagittal/oblique images should be parallel with the joint space and extend medially from the glenoid cavity laterally to the bicipital groove.

AXIAL IMAGES

A coronal image is used to determine the range of axial images. The range of axial images should extend from the acromion to the inferior aspect of the joint capsule (Fig. 23-5).

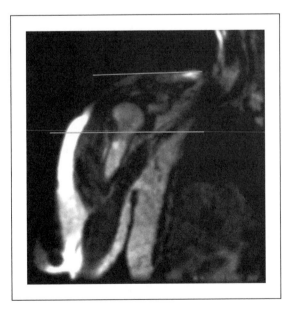

FIGURE 23-5

A coronal image is used to determine the range of axial images. The range of axial images should extend from the acromion to the inferior aspect of the joint capsule.

LONG BONE

Elective minimum required is 3.

Common Indications

- Evaluation of abnormalities involving the bony and soft tissue of long bones

Imaging Considerations

Imaging is completed with a surface coil. The patient position is dependent on the region of interest. If the proximal humerus is the area of question, the patient should be in a supine position with arms placed along the sides of the patient. If the area of interest is in the distal portion of the humerus or forearm, the patient should be in the prone position with the affected arm extended in the swimmer's position. The nonaffected arm should be placed along the side of the patient. If the patient is unable to assume the prone position, the supine position is adequate. For imaging of the lower long bones, the patient should be positioned supine with the area of interest entering the bore of the magnet first. Image weighting protocols can be customized to demonstrate the area of interest with consideration to scan time. Paramagnetic contrast medium is used per facility requirements. An accurate explanation of the examination process, with consideration of patient comfort, will reduce voluntary motion during the imaging process.

Patient Preparations

The surface coil should be placed lengthwise and parallel with the long bone. Align the patient so the affected long bone is close to the magnetic isocenter as possible. Measurement of the offset distance should be compensated for before imaging. If the patient is in the prone position, the longitudinal alignment light should be along the midline of the long bone. The horizontal alignment light should pass through the midline of the surface coil or midway between the superior and inferior border of the long bone. Place padding as needed to position the long bone with alignment light to avoid offset imaging. To minimize flow artifacts, the use of saturation pulses may be considered.

Imaging Protocols

The localizer image should include the entire long bone extending from the inferior to superior border. A coronal localizer should be used when evaluating lesions in the right to left axis, whereas a sagittal localizer should be used when evaluating lesions in the anterior to posterior axis.

SAGITTAL IMAGES

A coronal localizer image is used to determine the range of sagittal images. The range of sagittal images should extend from the medial to lateral borders of the long bone or region of interest.

CORONAL IMAGES

A sagittal image is used to determine the range of coronal images. The range of coronal images should extend from the anterior to posterior borders of the long bone or region of interest.

ELBOW

Mandatory minimum required is 4: This includes four examinations of the elbow, wrist, or hand in any combination.

Common Indications

- Evaluation of abnormalities involving the bony and soft tissue of the elbow

Imaging Considerations

Imaging is completed with either a flexible coil, two 5-in. circular coils, or extremity coil. The flexible coil should be attached without overlapping the coil. When using the 5-in. circular coils, they should be placed parallel to the elbow with both coils facing each other. The coils are centered to the elbow joint or the area of interest. When using the extremity coil, place the coil on the magnet end of the table. The patient is positioned prone, in a swimmer's position. The extremity coil should be centered on the elbow or affected area. Position the unaffected arm along the side of the patient. Image weighting protocols can be customized to demonstrate the area of interest within the elbow with consideration of scan time. Paramagnetic contrast medium is used per facility requirements. An accurate explanation of the examination process, with consideration of patient comfort, will reduce voluntary motion during the imaging process.

Patient Preparations

The patient's position is dependent on the patient's ability and on the specific coil used. Placement of padding to assist in centering the elbow within the coil as well as the magnetic isocenter may be necessary. Try and align the patient so the affected elbow is close to the magnetic isocenter as possible. Padding placed posterior to the patient's affected arm will aid in positioning the arm close to the

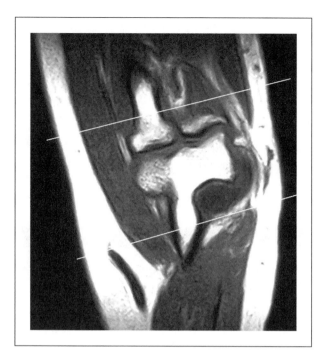

FIGURE 23-6

The coronal localizer image is used to determine the range of axial images. Obliquity of images may be necessary to achieve true planar images. The amount of obliquity is dependent on the positioning of the patient's arm. The range of axial images should extend through the joint or region of interest.

isocenter. Measurement of offset distance should be compensated for before imaging. The longitudinal alignment light should pass midway between the humeral condyles. The horizontal alignment light should pass through the humeral condyles. To minimize flow artifacts, the use of saturation pulses may be considered.

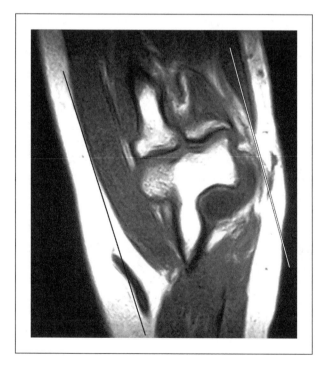

FIGURE 23-7

The same coronal localizer image is used to determine the range of oblique/sagittal images. Oblique/sagittal images should extend through the joint or region of interest.

Imaging Protocols

The coronal localizer image should include both the distal humerus and the proximal forearm.

AXIAL IMAGES

The coronal localizer image is used to determine the range of axial images. Obliquity of images may be necessary to achieve true planar images. The amount of obliquity is dependent on the positioning of the patient's arm. The range of axial images should extend through the joint or region of interest (Fig. 23-6).

SAGITTAL IMAGES

The same coronal localizer image is used to determine the range of oblique/sagittal images. Oblique/sagittal images should extend through the joint or region of interest (Fig. 23-7).

WRIST AND HAND

Mandatory minimum required is 4: This includes four examinations made of elbow, wrist, or hand in any combination.

Common Indications

- Visualization of scapholunate and scaphotriquetral ligaments
- Assessment of wrist pain of unknown origin
- Diagnosis of carpal tunnel syndrome

Imaging Considerations

Imaging of the wrist is completed with a choice of a dedicated wrist coil, round surface coil, single- or double-surface coils, or flexible coil. The flexible coil should be attached without overlapping of coil. Placement of padding to assist in centering the coil may be necessary. The wrist is usually scanned in the prone position; however, depending on the patient's ability, the wrist can be scanned in a lateral position with the thumb pointed up. Patient positioning is dependent on the type of coil selected. Image weighting protocols can be customized to demonstrate the area of interest with consideration of scan time. Paramagnetic contrast medium is used per facility requirements. An accurate explanation of the examination process, with consideration of patient comfort, will reduce voluntary motion during the imaging process.

Patient Preparations

The dedicated wrist coil should be attached at the head end of the examination table. The patient is placed in the prone position with the affected wrist extended over the head. The wrist is centered within the wrist coil and placed palm down or in a true lateral position with the thumb pointed up. The top half of the wrist coil should be locked down after alignment of the wrist to the isocenter of the coil.

When using the round surface coil, it should be placed over the center of the affected wrist. The patient should assume a prone position, head first, with the affected wrist placed prone and extended superior to the patient's head. The patient should form a fist with the affected hand to align the wrist parallel to the examination table.

When using a single surface coil, the technologist should place the coil on the dorsal side of the patient's affected wrist. If using two surface coils, the technologist should place one coil on the dorsal surface and the other coil on the ventral surface of the affected wrist. In both cases, the coil should be centered over the carpal bones. In the case of the single surface coil, the patient should assume a prone position, head first, with the affected wrist placed prone and extended superior to the patient's head. The patient should keep the affected hand in the prone position and extended superior to the patient's head. When using the dual surface coils, the patient should assume a supine position with the affected arm placed along the patient's side with the palm-side down.

The flexible coil is another option available to the technologist. The flexible coil should not be overlapped on itself. The patient is in the supine position during the examination with the affected arm placed along the side. The wrist is placed in a true lateral position with the hand parallel to the examination table.

Try and align the patient so that the affected wrist or hand is as close to the magnetic isocenter as possible. The horizontal alignment light should pass through the radial styloid process, whereas the longitudinal light passes through the center of the wrist joint. Padding placed around the forearm and shoulder will aid in positioning the wrist as close to the isocenter as possible, as well as minimizing motion artifacts. To minimize flow artifacts, the use of saturation pulses may be considered.

Imaging Protocols

The sagittal localizer image should extend inferiorly from the distal forearm through the carpals.

AXIAL IMAGES

A sagittal localizer image is used to determine the range of axial images. Axial images should range from inferior to superior surface of all carpals (Fig. 23-8).

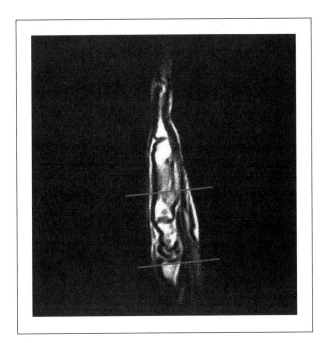

FIGURE 23-8

A sagittal localizer image is used to determine the range of axial images. Axial images should range from inferior to superior surface of all carpals.

CORONAL IMAGES

A sagittal localizer image is used to determine the range of coronal images. Oblique/coronal images should be completed per radiologist's request. Images should range from the anterior to posterior surface of the wrist and should have a sufficient FOV to include the distal forearm and distal border of carpals (Fig. 23-9).

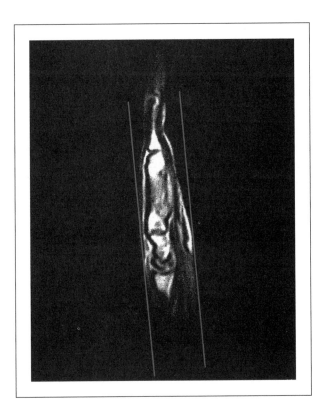

FIGURE 23-9

A sagittal localizer image is used to determine the range of coronal images. Oblique/coronal images should be completed per radiologist's request. Images should range from the anterior to posterior surface of the wrist and should have a sufficient FOV to include the distal forearm and distal border of carpals.

PELVIC GIRDLE

Elective minimum required is 3.

Common Indications

- Visualization of bladder, rectum, and urogenital tract
- Localization of undescended testicles
- Diagnosis of carcinoma of cervix, bladder, prostate, or rectum

Imaging Considerations

Pelvic imaging can be completed with the body coil or dedicated pelvic array coil. The pelvic coil should extend from the iliac crest through the symphysis. Image weighting protocols can be customized to demonstrate the area of interest within the pelvis with consideration of scan time. Paramagnetic contrast medium is used per facility requirements. An accurate explanation of the examination process, with consideration of patient comfort, will reduce voluntary motion during the imaging process.

Patient Preparations

The patient is placed feet first and supine on the examination table. The patient is positioned with the midsagittal plane aligned parallel with the longitudinal positioning light. Placing padding posterior to the patient's knees will reduce pressure in the area of the lumbar spine as well as flatten the pelvic area against the examination table. The horizontal alignment light should pass midway between the iliac crest and symphysis pubis. Foam pads and restraining straps should be positioned as needed. The patient's arms should be placed above the pelvis or along the sides of the patient. To minimize flow artifacts, the use of peripheral gating or saturation pulses may be considered. Pelvic motion can be reduced with compression or by instructing the patient to concentrate on breathing from the chest and upper abdomen without pelvic movement.

Imaging Protocols

The coronal localizer image should include the area from umbilicus to inferior pelvic border. The FOV should be adequate to include both lateral borders of the abdomen. Axial and sagittal images are determined by the coronal localizer image.

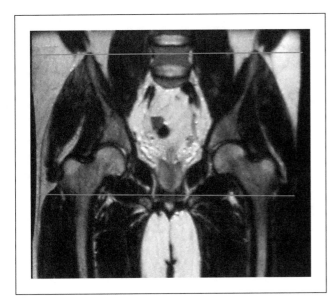

FIGURE 23-10

A coronal localizer image is used to determine the range of axial images. The range of axial images should extend from the iliac crest through the pelvic floor. The FOV is large enough to include the entire transverse image of the pelvis.

AXIAL IMAGES

A coronal localizer image is used to determine the range of axial images. The range of axial images should extend from the iliac crest through the pelvic floor. The FOV is large enough to include the entire transverse image of the pelvis (Fig. 23-10).

SAGITTAL IMAGES

An axial image is used to determine the range of sagittal images. Sagittal images can be taken from lateral border to opposite lateral border of the pelvis or through the specific area of interest. Sagittal

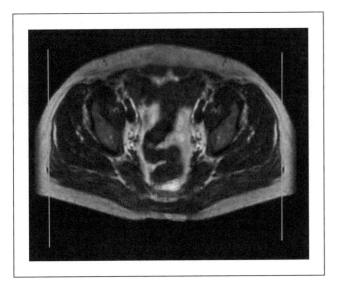

FIGURE 23-11

An axial image is used to determine the range of sagittal images. Sagittal images can be taken from lateral border to opposite lateral border of the pelvis or through the specific area of interest. Sagittal images are useful in evaluation of midline structures such as uterus, cervix, and vagina.

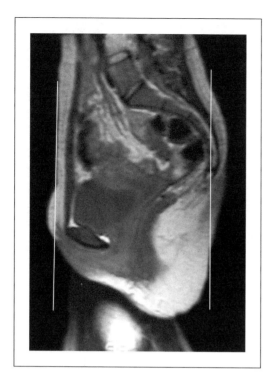

FIGURE 23-12

A sagittal image is used to determine the range of coronal images. Coronal images should extend from the anterior border of the symphysis pubis to the coccyx. The FOV should be large enough to include the iliac crest and symphysis pubis.

images are useful in evaluation of midline structures such as the uterus, cervix, and vagina (Fig. 23-11).

CORONAL IMAGES

A sagittal image is used to determine the range of coronal images. Coronal images should extend from the anterior border of the symphysis pubis to the coccyx. The FOV should be large enough to include the iliac crest and symphysis pubis. Coronal images are used to evaluate the pelvic sidewall for invasion in cases of uterine or cervical carcinoma (Fig. 23-12).

HIP

Mandatory minimum required is 4.

Common Indications

- Rule out labral tears
- Evaluation of unexplained hip pain

Imaging Considerations

Pelvic imaging can be completed with the body coil or dedicated pelvic array coil. The pelvic coil should extend from the iliac crest through the symphysis. Image weighting protocols can be customized to demonstrate the area of interest within the pelvis with consideration of scan time. Paramagnetic contrast medium is used per facility requirements. An accurate explanation of the examination process, with consideration of patient comfort, will reduce voluntary motion during the imaging process.

Patient Preparations

When using the pelvic coil, place the coil around pelvis with hip joints located in center of coil. When using the pelvic coil or body coil, place the patient supine, feet-first into the magnet. The patient's body should be aligned so that the midsagittal portion of the body is parallel with the middle of the examination table. The patient's arms should be placed along the sides or across the upper abdomen. Immobilization straps can be used to provide support for the arms. The patient's legs should be straight with the feet pointed up. Use of tape around the patient's feet and positioning padding should be considered. The horizontal alignment light should pass through the hip joint. If one hip is to be imaged, try and position the patient so the affected hip is close to the magnetic isocenter. To minimize flow artifacts, the use of saturation pulses may be considered.

Imaging Protocols

The coronal localizer image should include the pelvis from lateral to lateral border and extend inferior from the iliac crest.

CORONAL IMAGES

An axial image is used to determine the range of coronal images. Coronal images should be parallel to the femoral neck and from the posterior to anterior borders of the femoral head. The FOV of each

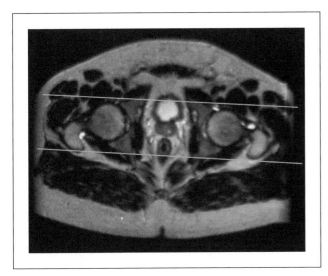

FIGURE 23-13

An axial image is used to determine the range of coronal images. Coronal images should be parallel to the femoral neck and from the posterior to anterior borders of the femoral head. The FOV of each image should include the proximal margin of the femoral shaft to the greater sciatic notch.

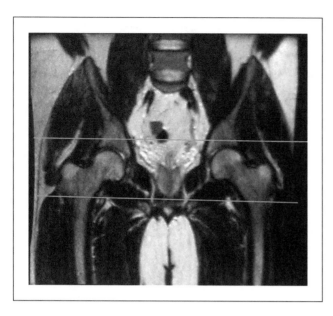

FIGURE 23-14

A coronal image is used to determine the range of axial images. The range of axial images should extend through the hip joint or region of interest.

image should include the proximal margin of the femoral shaft to the greater sciatic notch (Fig. 23-13).

AXIAL IMAGES

A coronal image is used to determine the range of axial images. The range of axial images should extend through the hip joint or region of interest (Fig. 23-14).

KNEE

Mandatory minimum required is 6.

Common Indications

- Evaluation of patella and patella tracking
- Visualization of knee disorders, including bony tumors
- Visualization and assessment of meniscus and cruciate tears

Imaging Considerations

Imaging is completed with a flexible coil or designated extremity coil. The flexible coil should be attached without overlapping of coil. Placement of padding to assist in centering the coil may be necessary. Padding should be placed under patient's feet to comfortably extend, without hyperextending, the knee. The patient is positioned supine and feet first, with the arms placed along the patient's side or across the lower abdomen. Image weighting protocols can be customized to demonstrate the area of interest within the knee with consideration of scan time. Paramagnetic contrast medium is used per facility requirements. An accurate explanation of the examination process, with consideration of patient comfort, will reduce voluntary motion during the imaging process.

Patient Preparations

Attach the flexible coil while centering it over the affected knee. Place the knee close to the magnetic isocenter. Do not allow the coil to touch the sides of the bore. Use of thermal resistant padding may be necessary between the coil and bore surface. When using the designated extremity coil, place the coil on the end of the table that will enter the magnet first. Place the affected knee in the bottom half of the coil, while at the same time aligning the knee to the coil. Latch the top half of the coil after centering is completed. When using either coil, the knee should be rotated according to scan protocol to visualize the desired ligament. The affected knee should be placed with the longitudinal alignment light running through the longitudinal axis of the leg. The horizontal alignment light should pass through the apex of the patella. It is important to place padding on the unaffected knee to improve the patient's comfort. To minimize flow artifacts, the use of saturation pulses may be considered.

Imaging Protocols

The coronal, sagittal, or axial localizer image should display the knee joint in the center of the FOV.

CORONAL IMAGES

A sagittal localizer image is used to determine the range of coronal images. The coronal images should be placed with knee joint centered

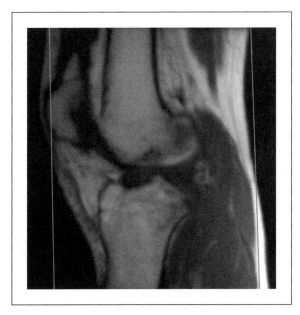

FIGURE 23-15

A sagittal localizer image is used to determine the range of coronal images. The coronal images should be placed with knee joint centered in the FOV. Coronal images should be from the posterior skin surface and extend to the anterior surface of the patella. The borders of the image should include the proximal patellar border and proximal tibia.

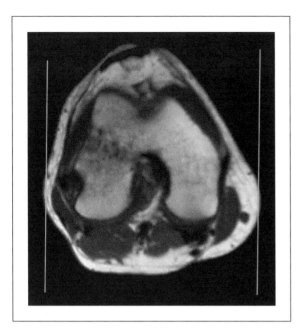

FIGURE 23-16

An axial image is used to determine the range of sagittal images. Sagittal images should be placed with knee joint centered in the FOV. Sagittal images should be from the lateral to medial skin surface of the knee. The borders of the image should include the lateral condyles of the femur as well as the proximal tibia.

in the FOV. Coronal images should be from the posterior skin surface and extend to the anterior surface of the patella. The borders of the image should include the proximal patellar border and proximal tibia (Fig. 23-15).

SAGITTAL IMAGES

An axial image is used to determine the range of sagittal images. Sagittal images should be placed with the knee joint centered in the FOV. Sagittal images should be from the lateral to medial skin surface of the knee. The borders of the image should include the lateral condyles of the femur as well as the proximal tibia (Fig. 23-16).

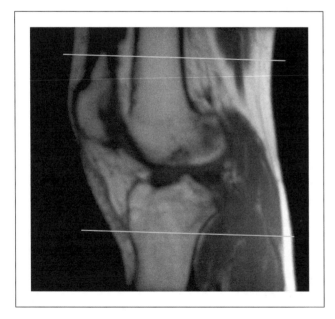

FIGURE 23-17

The sagittal image is used to determine the range of axial images. The range of axial images should extend through the region of interest or as determined by imaging facility and radiologist preference.

AXIAL IMAGES

A sagittal image is used to determine the range of axial images. The range of axial images should extend through the region of interest or as determined by imaging facility and radiologist preference (Fig. 23-17).

ANKLE AND FOOT

Mandatory minimum required is 4.

Common Indications

- Visualization of tendons, muscles, and soft tissue abnormalities
- Diagnosis of bony tumors and trauma

Imaging Considerations

Imaging is completed with either a flexible coil, designated extremity coil, or head coil. The flexible coil should be attached without overlapping the coil. Placement of padding to assist in centering the coil may be necessary. The patient's arms are placed along the sides of the patient. Image weighting protocols can be customized to demonstrate the area of interest within the foot or ankle, with consideration of scan time. Paramagnetic contrast medium is used per facility requirements. An accurate explanation of the examination process, with consideration of patient comfort, will reduce voluntary motion during the imaging process.

Patient Preparations

The patient is positioned supine and feet first into the magnet. When using the flexible coil, place the coil around the ankle, with mesh openings on the lateral and medial borders of ankle. Use of immobilization straps to align and stabilize feet should be considered. When using the designated extremity coil, have the patient slightly flex the knee and place the lower leg over a cushion or padding to allow the foot to lie in the bottom half of the coil. Align the patient so the affected ankle is close to the magnetic isocenter. The head coil is another alternative when imaging the ankles. Place both of the patient's feet within the head coil. Allow the patient to relax both legs parallel with the examination table. Center the anatomy within the head coil. When using any coil, use padding in pressure areas of the body to ensure patient comfort and reduction of motion. The longitudinal alignment light should lie midline to the affected ankle. The horizontal alignment light should pass midline of the affected foot. To minimize flow artifacts, the use of saturation pulses may be considered.

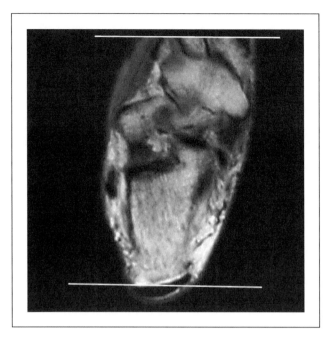

FIGURE 23-18

A coronal localizer image is used to determine the range of axial images from the plantar to dorsal borders of the foot. The angle of obliquity is determined by the positioning of the foot and ankle.

Imaging Protocols

The coronal localizer image should include the distal tibia to plantar surface of the foot. The coronal localizer is used to determine the sagittal and axial images.

AXIAL IMAGES

A coronal localizer image is used to determine the range of axial images from the plantar to dorsal borders of the foot. The angle of obliquity is determined by the positioning of the foot and ankle (Fig. 23-18).

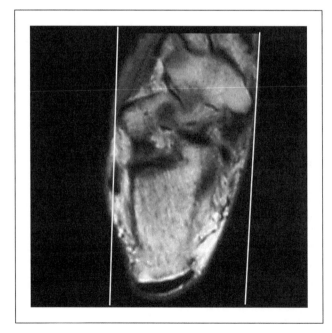

FIGURE 23-19

A coronal localizer image is used to determine the range of sagittal images. Images should range from border to opposite border of the ankle. The image should include both tarsals and metatarsals.

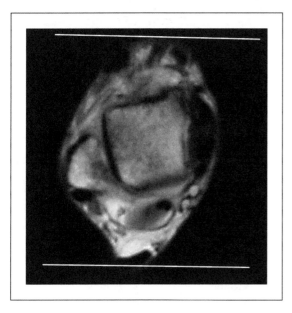

FIGURE 23-20

An axial image is used to determine the range of coronal images. Images should range from border to opposite border of the ankle. The image should include both tarsals and metatarsals.

SAGITTAL IMAGES

A coronal localizer image is used to determine the range of sagittal images. Images should range from border to opposite border of the ankle. The image should include both tarsals and metatarsals (Fig. 23-19).

CORONAL IMAGES

An axial image is used to determine the range of coronal images. Images should range from border to opposite border of the ankle. The image should include both tarsals and metatarsals (Fig. 23-20).

VASCULAR IMAGING OF THE LOWER LIMBS

Elective minimum required is 3.

Common Indications

- Evaluation of peripheral vascular network of the lower limbs
- Assessment of normal vasculature before coronary bypass surgery

Imaging Considerations

Imaging is completed with the body, flexible surface, or extremity coil. The surface or extremity coil is used for imaging the vascular structures of the feet and lower legs. The body coil is used to image the femur and pelvic imaging of the vascular network. The flexible coil should be attached without overlapping the coil. Placement of padding and immobilization straps to assist in centering of coil may be necessary. The patient is positioned supine and feet first into the magnet. The arms are placed along the side or across the upper abdomen. If vascular imaging of the legs is performed, the patient's legs should be extended flat. If vascular imaging of the feet is performed, the feet should be flat on the coil, with support padding placed posterior to the knees. Image weighting protocols can be customized to demonstrate the area of interest within the lower limb with consideration of scan time. Paramagnetic contrast medium is used per facility requirements. An accurate explanation of the examination process, with consideration of patient comfort, will reduce voluntary motion during the imaging process.

Patient Preparations

When using a 2D time of flight imaging technique, numerous axial images are acquired through the area of interest. The patient is positioned so the longitudinal light runs through the midsagittal portion of the patient. The horizontal alignment light should pass through the center of the region of interest. Overlapping of the image ranges by 2.5 cm is important because the entire lower limb is not displayed in the same FOV. Use of localization markers will aid in the patient positioning of the different ranges. To minimize flow artifacts, the use of saturation pulses may be considered.

Imaging Protocols

The localizer image should include the area of interest extending from superior to inferior borders of coil and lateral and medial borders of anatomic part. The images should include the specific area of interest. The slices should be continuous or gathered in a volume of information at one given time. The process of 2D time of flight MRA is used to gather the information. After the examination, the technologist can reconstruct the information into desired imaging planes.

KINEMATIC STUDIES

Elective minimum required is 3.

Common Indications

- Assessment of internal meniscal derangement

Imaging Considerations

Studies of the temporomandibular joints (TMJs) will frequently include a complete head examination. Imaging is completed with dual 3-in. coils. The patient is placed head first and supine on the examination table. The patient's arms should lay along the side. The designated dual 3-in. coils should be placed as close to the surface of the patient as possible without touching. Both joints are imaged simultaneously. Image weighting protocols can be customized to demonstrate the area of interest with consideration of scan time. Paramagnetic contrast medium is used per facility requirements. An accurate explanation of the examination process, with consideration of patient comfort, will reduce voluntary motion during the imaging process.

Patient Preparations

The patient is positioned with the midsagittal plane aligned parallel with the longitudinal positioning light. Placing padding posterior to the patient's knees will reduce pressure in the area of the lumbar spine and increase patient comfort. The horizontal alignment light should pass through the level of the TMJ, centered within the coil. Foam pads and restraining straps should be positioned as needed. The patient's arms should be placed across the abdomen or along the patient's sides. Use of saturation pulses and triggering is normally not necessary for TMJ imaging. Instruct the patient of proper timing for opening and closing of mouth before imaging. Use of a mouth-opening device may be necessary. The kinematic TMJ protocol begins with the mouth closed, then repeat the same locations in incremental steps for different mouth positions.

Imaging Protocols

The axial localizer image should include the entire area of the head.

SAGITTAL/OBLIQUE IMAGES

An axial localizer image is used to determine the range of sagittal/oblique images. The range of sagittal/oblique images should extend from the lateral to medial border of the temporomandibular joint.

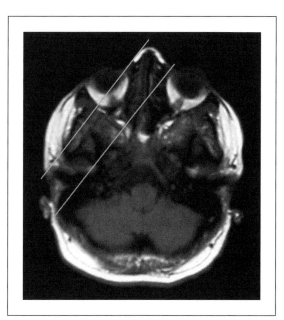

FIGURE 23-21

An axial localizer image is used to determine the range of sagittal/oblique images. The range of sagittal/oblique images should extend from the lateral to medial border of the temporomandibular joint. Slices should be angled perpendicular to the mandibular condyles. Both temporomandibular joints can be displayed on each image.

Slices should be angled perpendicular to the mandibular condyles. Both temporomandibular joints can be displayed on each image (Fig. 23-21).

CORONAL IMAGES

An axial image is used to determine the range of coronal images. For coronal images, slices should be aligned parallel with the temporomandibular joint. The range of images should extend through the area of interest (Fig. 23-22).

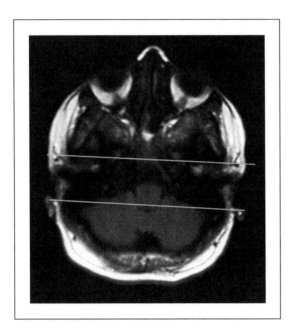

FIGURE 23-22

An axial image is used to determine the range of coronal images. For coronal images, slices should be aligned parallel with the temporomandibular joint. The range of images should extend through the area of interest.

CHAPTER 24

Advanced MR Imaging Procedures

Elective minimum required is 3.

Common Indications

To demonstrate the quality of blood supply of the brain tissues and other highly vascular organs such as the heart, kidneys, liver, and spleen.

Imaging Considerations

Perfusion is the amount of blood flow through 1 g of tissue. Perfusion imaging is a method to measure the quality vascular supply to tissue. This is inherently related to a person's metabolic activity and, therefore, is a method to assess the activity of the specific area of interest. The principle of perfusion imaging is the measurement of the signal generated from the hydrogen atoms present in the arterial blood supply.

Methods of visualization include the application of saturation pulses, use of an inversion recovery pulse sequence, or the introduction of injectable contrast medium. Perfusion images should be generated by using ultrafast imaging sequences. Using ultrafast acquisition techniques, images can be attained before, during, and after bolus injections.

As a contrast agent, gadolinium will reduce the T2 and T2* decay times. The reduced signal decay is used to evaluate the blood volume changes over time. Creation of a cerebral blood volume map is completed by combining time intensity curves for multiple images during and after the injection of gadolinium. It has been found that malignancy of neoplasms is associated with the increase of perfusion or metabolic activity. On a cerebral vascular map, the areas of low perfusion will seem hypointense. These areas have been associated with stroke. Areas with a high amount of perfusion on a cerebral vascular map will have a hyperintense appearance and have been associated with malignancies.

DIFFUSION IMAGING

Elective minimum required is 3.

Common Indications

- For diagnosis of stroke
- Demonstration of reversible and irreversible ischemic lesions
- Discrimination of salvageable tissues before therapeutic intervention

Imaging Considerations

Diffusion is the movement of molecules due to random thermal motion. This molecular motion is restricted by the natural boundaries of membranes and macromolecules. There is a critical time during the early stages of stroke that cells absorb water from the extracellular space. At this point, the process of diffusion is restricted and the diffusion rate reduced in this specific area. This event occurs after the onset of ischemia but before infarct or permanent tissue damage. Timing of a diffusion study is critical because reduced diffusion occurs several days after the beginning of a stroke.

When using a spin echo sequence in normal imaging, the use of a refocusing pulse will rephase the hydrogen atoms that are present during the transmission of the refocusing process. In the event that the hydrogen atoms move out of this designated area through the process of diffusion, the signal will be reduced. When echo planar imaging is used in diffusion imaging, two gradient pulses are used. The principle behind this is the atoms which do not diffuse will cancel out the affects of the two gradient pulses and result in a hyperintense signal. The atoms that diffused will experience a phase shift when the two gradient pulses are used. The gradient pulses can be applied to the $x, y,$ or z gradients to determine the direction of diffusion. Diffusion imaging uses similar gradient systems as MRA. The use of ultrafast techniques such as spin echo, echo planar imaging (spin echo EPI or SE EPI), and the use of strong gradients will reduce motion artifacts created by phase changes.

FUNCTIONAL MRI

Elective minimum required is 3.

Common Indications

- Acquiring images of the brain during activity, stimulus, or rest
- Evaluation of stroke, epilepsy, pain, and behavioral problems

Imaging Considerations

Before understanding functional MRI (fMRI), it is necessary to have a basic understanding of the involvement of blood. Hemoglobin is the iron-containing pigment of the red blood cell. Hemoglobin functions by carrying oxygen from the lungs to the tissues of the body. The amount of hemoglobin present in males will usually range from 14 to 18 g/100 mL of blood. The average adult female has a hemoglobin level from 12 to 16 g/100 mL of blood. When hemoglobin combines with oxygen, the resulting compound is oxyhemoglobin. The oxyhemoglobin state reacts to the magnetic influences in a diamagnetic manner and, therefore, suppresses the magnetic properties of the iron. When oxygen is not present with hemoglobin, the result is deoxyhemoglobin. Deoxyhemoglobin reacts to the magnetic influences in a paramagnetic manner. The paramagnetic state of deoxyhemoglobin creates an inhomogeneous magnetic field and increases the amount of $T2^*$ decay in the specific areas containing deoxyhemoglobin.

When the patient is at rest, the mixture of deoxyhemoglobin and oxyhemoglobin is equal. With activity, the metabolism increases and the level of oxyhemoglobin decreases in the brain. The decrease in oxyhemoglobin will cause the cerebral vascular system to increase the blood flow to the activated area. Blood oxygenation increases to specific areas during brain activity. Increased blood flow is present in areas of the visual cortex during seeing activities. There is also an increase in flow to the motor cortex during simple finger-tapping activities. This dependency of oxygenated blood is termed "blood oxygenation level–dependent" (BOLD). Functional MRI uses BOLD by analyzing the magnetic susceptibility of oxyhemoglobin and deoxyhemoglobin.

Functional MR imaging uses normal images taken without activity, followed by the images with brain activity. This activity process can be simple as an oscillating light in the patient's eyes. The second set of images are then subtracted, demonstrating the functional brain activity that results from the increased blood flow to the activated cortex. The signal from the deoxyhemoglobin results in an increase in

297

signal intensity. The effects of BOLD occur rapidly and, therefore, justify rapid imaging sequences such as EPI.

ECHO PLANAR IMAGING APPLICATIONS

Elective minimum required is 3.

Common Indications

- Acquiring images with a minimal amount of acquisition time
- Reduction of scan time per patient will reduce the likelihood of motion
- Functional imaging of the brain
- Dynamic imaging of the kidney
- Imaging fast-moving structures such as the heart

Imaging Considerations

One of the goals of MRI is to achieve the best possible spatial and contrast resolution in the shortest amount of time. Like many things in life, achieving all of these goals equally is not possible, and MRI is no different in this aspect. The result is a collaborative effort of acceptable image quality in a reasonable amount of time. Echo planar imaging (EPI) is currently the fastest method of acquiring information. EPI is frequently divided into two subdivisions, spin echo EPI and gradient echo EPI. Before discussing the mapping of information of EPI images, it is necessary to explain the process of image mapping in conventional spin echo imaging.

Once the acquired spatial frequencies are attained, they must be coded and decoded within a reconstruction portion of the computer. This coding and filing method is termed "k-space" filing. In conventional spin echo imaging for each line in the k-space file, the phase-encoding gradient is applied. In conventional spin echo, only one line of k-space is filled during each radio frequency. If 256 lines of k-space need to be filled to create an image, there will be an equal amount of phase encoding. In addition, each line of k-space is filled from the same direction such as from left to right across the k-space file. If the process takes 100 ms and there are 256 phase encodings, then it will take 25.6 s to acquire one image. This process is very time consuming and does not always allow for the mobility of blood, CSF, or patient motion. Options to reduce the scan time in conventional imaging are to reduce the length of repetition time, or to fill more than one line of k-space per repetition time.

The principal idea of EPI is to fill all the k-space lines in one given pulse of the submitted radio frequency. During the pulse sequence, the frequency-encoding gradient is oscillating from a positive to negative polarity. When the frequency-encoding gradient is influenced by the positive polarity, it will fill the k-space file from left to right. When the frequency-encoding gradient polarity is reversed to the negative direction, the k-space file will fill from right to left. The phase-encoding gradient is momentarily activated between each frequency-encoding period. This method of momentarily activating the phase-encoding gradient, also referred to as a "phase blip," will advance the k-space line to the next line of k-space. This method will allow each line of k-space to be filled in an opposite direction, as from left to right, then the next line is filled from right to left. This is a more efficient manner of completing the spatial frequency-encoding instead of that of conventional spin echo imaging.

EPI uses rapidly oscillating gradients to spatially encode the MRI signal. In conventional MR imaging, repetition time (TR) represents each line of k-space filled, with all the lines of k-space being filled during each repetition time. With EPI the TR now represents the time between each completed image. To produce an image in a few milliseconds, the MR unit is required to have very strong gradients that have capabilities to be switched in polarity during a radio sequence.

Clinical Applications of EPI

The principal advantage of EPI is the ability to acquire an image in times from 50 to 100 ms. Brain imaging can be completed with the use of EPI. EPI will reduce or remove motion artifacts completely. Typical applications include functional studies of the brain such as cerebral blood volume (CBV) mapping, perfusion, and diffusion imaging. With the ability to image faster, there is now an absence of movement. Dynamic imaging of the kidney to quantify physiology and renal artery stenosis is showing promise with the use of EPI. EPI is also useful at imaging fast-moving structures such as the heart. Actual images of the heart frozen in time demonstrate cardiac hemodynamics with and without contrast agents. The visualization of valve leaflets and valvular insufficiency is now possible with the use of real-time EPI. This process can create up to 10 images per second.

Artifacts of EPI

Artifacts consist of chemical shift artifact, which makes it necessary to use some sort of fat saturation to reduce the intensity from fat.

Biological Concerns

The constant polarity shifting of the frequency-encoding gradient produces sounds measuring from 90 to 110 db. This is one of the unfortunate affects of EPI and currently is addressed with the use of commercial-quality earplugs to attenuate the sound. One of the concerns of EPI is the physiologic stimulation created by the rapidly changing magnetic field. The rapidly changing magnetic field may produce a nerve stimulation, leading to muscle contraction.

3D VOLUME REFORMATION

Elective minimum required is 3.

Common Indications

- Acquiring entire volumes of information during one acquisition time, which can be later reconstructed in any plane at a variety of slice thicknesses
- Increasing spatial resolution of an image
- Three-dimensional magnetic resonance angiography

Imaging Considerations

When an image is generated in a single slice format, it is termed two-dimensional imaging. The Fourier transformation process is used to transform the spatial frequencies into a computer generated two-dimensional (2D-FT) image. Two-dimensional Fourier transformation encodes the information by using the three axes during the application of the pulse sequence. The slice-select gradient is activated simultaneously when the radio frequency (RF) pulse is transmitted into the specific body part. The phase-encoding gradient is applied between the RF pulse and the generation of the signal. The frequency-encoding gradient is applied simultaneously during the signal generation. This process ensures the proper assigning of signal information into the proper k-space file. The encoding of information in the 2D-FT process is repeated until all the lines of the k-space file are filled. Therefore, if 256 lines of k-space are to be filled, there will be 256 phase encodings, slice-select gradient applications, and frequency-encoding gradients. The scan time in 2D-FT is a product of repetition time, the number of phase encodings, and the number of excitations.

Three-dimensional imaging also uses the Fourier transformation process and is thus termed "3D-FT" imaging. The 3D information is initially gathered by transmitting the radio frequency into a volume of tissue, such as the entire volume of brain tissue. Instead of acquiring the information for one slice of information, as in 2D-FT, the 3D-FT stores all the information from the volume of tissue. 3D-FT does not use the slice-select gradient simultaneously with the transmitted RF pulse. Because the slice-select gradient is not used, the entire volume of tissue is excited by the RF pulse. The frequency-encoding gradient is activated simultaneously as the echo is generated. The phase-encoding gradient is turned in both of the remaining axes to encode the information in the proper k-space file. Because 3D-FT does not apply the slice-select gradient and a volume of tissue is excited by the RF pulse, the addition of an extra phase-encoding gradient is used in the third axis to ensure proper coding of information. Therefore, the scan time of 3D-FT is considerably longer than that of 2D-FT. The scan time for a 3D-FT image is the product of the number of both phase encodings, the number of excitations, and the repetition time. After the acquisition of 3D-FT information, the patient can leave while the technologist reconstructs the volume of information into the desired imaging planes. Images can be reconstructed in slice thicknesses to as little as 1 mm. 3D-FT is useful in the imaging of anatomic images of the lumbar spine and pituitary, especially in areas where the use of T1-weighted images are sufficient. Spatial resolution is increased if the slice thickness will equal the width and height of each pixel. This process results in an isotropic voxel.

MULTIPLANAR REFORMATION

Elective minimum required is 3.

Common Indications

- Reformation of image data into any orthogonal or oblique plane
- Commonly used for musculoskeletal and vascular applications

Imaging Considerations

Multiplanar reformation (MPR) is a computer process that is completed after the gathering of a volume of information through 3D imaging. The 3D process gathers a block or volume of information when the RF pulse is introduced to the area of interest such as the entire head from superior to inferior aspect. This process occurs because the slice-encoding gradient is not applied during the pulse sequence. The MR computer uses the frequency-encoding gradient as in 2D imaging. Unlike 2D imaging, 3D imaging uses two phase gradients to encode the information. The first phase-encoding gradient is used similar to the 2D process but the second phase encoding is used for storing the image in the third, or volume, direction. The second-phase encoding process will be repeated as many times as the technologist requires slices of information; for example, if the technologist requests eight slices, there will be eight additional phase encodings in the slice direction of the volume of information.

When using the second phase-encoding process, the scan time in 3D volume imaging is considerably longer than that of 2D imaging. This is due to the addition of the phase encodings required in the slice direction. The scan time for 3D imaging is the product of repetition time, number of signal acquisitions, the number of phase lines within the matrix, and the number of slices to be reconstructed. To reduce the longer scan times required by 3D imaging, a gradient echo sequence is often used. The increase in signal to noise ratio (SNR) from 3D volume imaging makes the increase in scan time a sufficient trade-off. During 2D imaging, a slice of information is sampled. There is normally a gap between each additional slice to avoid the artifact from cross-excitation or cross-talk between consecutive slices. The process of MPR eliminates the problem of cross-talk and can use the 3D volume of information to reconstruct images with contiguous slices.

The image plane is divided into three dimensions, two of which are determined by the matrix. The matrix is a grid-type layout of the scan information. The field of view (FOV) will determine the height and width of the matrix. The number of pixels in each of the dimensions will determine the matrix size. The number and thickness of slices make up the volume portion of the gathered information and will determine the third dimension. Because the "pixel" makes up the height and width dimension and the slice thickness is responsible for the dimension of depth, we can now refer to the volume of information as a "voxel." If the matrix of 256 by 256 is selected, there will be 256 pixels in the frequency-encoding direction and 256 pixels in the phase-encoding direction. Until we know the height and width of the FOV, we cannot determine the size or area of each pixel. If the FOV is determined to be 260 mm in both height and width dimensions, then the height and width of each pixel can be determined by dividing the FOV by the matrix size (256). In this example, the pixel is equal to 1.015 mm in both the height and width dimensions. The pixels in the slice thickness dimension should be of equal size as the other two dimensions to retain optimal reconstruction quality. When the voxel is equal in all three dimensions, it is considered "isotropic." If the voxel is longer or shorter in the direction of slice thickness, the voxel will represent an oblong box as opposed to a perfect cube. The unequal voxel is referred to as "anisotropic." For optimal spatial resolution in any plane, the use of isotropic voxels is necessary.

After the 3D imaging process the patient is often removed from the MR unit. The technologist is able to complete MPR on the gathered image data. Images can be reconstructed into any orthogonal plane or obliquity. Some manufacturers have introduced the reconstruction process that allows for a curved reformatted view.

SPECTROSCOPY

Elective minimum required is 3.

Common Indications

- To perform in vivo analysis of pathology
- Evaluation of suspicious lesions of the brain by using a spectrographic display
- Comparisons of chemical compositions of *N*-acetyl aspartate, *N*-acetyl aspartate glutamate, choline-containing compounds,

creatine-containing compounds, myo-inositol, and glucose

Imaging Considerations

The basic idea of MRI is each element within our bodies has a unique resonance frequency at a given magnetic field strength. Because elements within the body combine to form molecules, each molecular structure will have a unique resonance frequency. *Chemical shift* is the term used to describe the differences in frequencies in molecules. The principle behind the chemical shift involves the electrons surrounding atoms. The electrons have their own rotation, which results in a magnetic field surrounding the electron. This small magnetic field can have a positive or negative influence on the nucleus of the atom and, thus, alters the precisional frequency of the atom. This small influence is enough to create a unique difference in each molecule. This difference is graphically displayed by a unique frequency shift in spectroscopy.

Spectroscopy is an available option to determine whether a suspicious lesion is healthy or abnormal tissue. Spectroscopy is completed after the normal brain scan. The cursor is placed over the region of interest within the brain. For spectroscopy information, a square display or "scan box" will appear on the viewing monitor. Placement of the scan box over the region of interest without containing pulsatile CSF in the ventricles or an area of lipids is important. The goal is to gather information from a homogenous sample of tissue. The region of interest is scanned, and the computer will graphically display the specific frequency-related material of the molecular composition of the tissue within the region of interest. Currently, the most popular chemical information is related to *N*-acetyl aspartate, *N*-acetyl aspartate glutamate, choline-containing compounds, creatine-containing compounds, myo-inositol, and glucose. All of these compounds have been found to differ from their normal spatial frequencies in abnormal tissues of the brain. Recent findings have shown *N*-acetyl aspartate (NAA) is located primarily within neurons and has the most characteristic change in abnormal tissue. NAA has allowed a functional aspect of the brain. Clinical applications for spectroscopy to the brain has shown promise in patients with HIV infection, AIDS, multiple sclerosis, epilepsy, Parkinson's disease, Alzheimer's disease, primary and metastatic brain tumors, hepatic encephalopathy, and stroke.

NONIMAGING AND QUALITY ASSURANCE PROCEDURES IN MRI

CHAPTER 25

Intravenous Injections of Contrast Medium

CONTRAST AGENT PREPARATION

Mandatory minimum required is 4.

Common Indications

- Evaluation of the blood-brain barrier
- Enhancement of tumors before and after operation
- Infection, infarction, and inflammation
- Post-traumatic lesions in the central nervous system
- Postoperative lumbar disk

Imaging Considerations

Approximately one-third of the MRI studies in the United States use contrast agents as a part of the normal procedure. Contrast agents used in MRI are currently based on the gadolinium atom. Gadolinium is considered a toxic "heavy metal," but when bound to diethylenetriamine pentaacetic acid or other chelate, it is safe for human use. Gadolinium is a paramagnetic substance and, therefore, influenced in a positive manner when placed in a magnetic field. Contrast agents in MRI are normally injected intravenously. Approximately 80% of the gadolinium agent will be excreted by the kidneys in 3 h, and 98% will be recovered by the feces and urine within 7 days. The side effects after the injection of gadolinium-based agents include a slight increase in bilirubin and blood iron. Less than 10% of the patients will experience mild headaches, 4% of the patients will experience nausea, 2% will experience vomiting, and less than 1% of the injections will result in rash. Patients should be properly screened, and the contrast agent package insert should always be reviewed before injection. Current changes in quantities and properties of contrast agents can be determined by reading the package insert.

There are currently no contraindications for the use of the FDA-approved paramagnetic contrast agents. There are, however, precautions concerning the use in patients with renal or hepatic impairment, patients who are breast feeding, patients with deoxygenated sickle erythrocytes, and patients younger than 18 years old. The paramagnetic contrast agents used in MRI require substantially less amounts in comparison to computed tomography or diagnostic radiography. Patient dose calculations are dependent on physician preference and manufacturer's recommendations. Recommended doses range from 0.2 mL/kg to a maximum dosage of 14 mL of contrast agent per patient. To ensure the complete injection of paramagnetic contrast agent, the technologist should follow the injection with a 5-mL of saline flush. Any unused portion of contrast agent should be immediately disposed of. Imaging should be completed within 1 h of the injection of the contrast agent.

Gadolinium-based contrast agents are designed to reduce the longitudinal relaxation (T1 times) of the tissue. By reducing the T1 time, an increased signal will result in the area where the contrast agent is present. T2 decay times will also be reduced, but at the current dose, T1 times will be more apparent. Contrast agents do not penetrate the normal blood-brain barrier; however, areas of abnormal vascularity or disruption of blood-brain barrier will allow for the accumulation of the contrast agent. With reduced T1 times, neoplasms, abscesses, and subacute infarcts will have a bright appearance; this is why gadolinium is considered a T1 enhancement agent. When using a gadolinium-based contrast agent, the total examination time will be increased because the additional contrast sequence has been added. Most protocols will call for the injection of contrast agent after the normal MR imaging protocol.

For examinations of the lumbar spine, differentiating between scar tissue and recurrent herniated disk becomes more apparent with injection of the paramagnetic contrast agent. The scar tissue initially will enhance, whereas the disk will not. However, after a 30-min delay, the disk will show signs of enhancement.

VENIPUNCTURE

Mandatory minimum required is 4.

This procedure may be simulated in those states or institutions where venipuncture by registered technologists is prohibited.

Common Indications

- Method of quick absorption of medication into the circulatory system
- Method of quick response for medication
- Alternative solution for drugs that cannot be given orally

Imaging Considerations

Intravenous injections are a method of introducing medications or contrast medium into the circulatory system. The response to the medication is rapid and can be the choice of administration when the drug is impalpable or the patient is unable orally to consume the drug. Not all clinical settings allow the registered technologist to start or inject intravenous contrast medium. Registered technologists permitted to inject intravenous drugs should familiarize themselves with facility standards. If the facility does not allow the registered technologist to start the infusion site, the technologists can assist the qualified personnel by organizing the necessary supplies for starting an infusion site.

It is prudent for the technologist to obtain the patient's vital signs before an intravenous injection. This method provides a baseline for comparison in the event of a sudden change to the patient's condition after injection of drugs or contrast medium. A drug administered intravenously will generate a rapid response; in addition, the drug cannot be retrieved once injected into the person. The technologist should never leave the patient after the administration of an intravenous drug or contrast agent. The patient should be visually and verbally monitored throughout the examination process.

Medical asepsis is mandatory for all drugs and contrast to be administered intravenously. Certain drugs can be given intravenously through an existing line, with consideration to the following factors:

- Facility specification
- Type of the preexisting line
- Type of drug present in the existing line
- Specific drug to be administered
- Amount of drug or contrast to be administered
- Rate at which the drug or contrast medium is to be administered

307

The same factors will determine the type and size of catheter to be used in the event a new intravenous site must be found. Drugs administered slowly, or of low viscosity, can be injected through a smaller gauge needle such as a 20- to 25-gauge needle. For drugs introduced over a long period of time and for drugs administered in large amounts (such as 250–1000 mL), consider using a 20-gauge needle to administer the drug. In addition, for the injection of very viscid drugs or contrast medium, consider the use of a larger bore needle. Most facilities prefer the use of a butterfly needle or venous or angiocatheters to administer drugs or contrast medium. The process and necessary supplies needed for starting an infusion site will vary slightly among facilities; the technologist should be familiar with the specific protocols.

VITAL SIGNS (BLOOD PRESSURE, PULSE, RESPIRATION, TEMPERATURE)

Mandatory minimum required is 4.

Common Indications

- When there is a change in the patient's condition
- Taken before and after any interventional or invasive diagnostic procedure

Imaging Considerations

Vital signs consist of measurements of the patient's current blood pressure, pulse, respiration, and temperature values. These rates are compared with the rate or value of the average person in the same age category or preferable to the patient's previous values. The technologist should be aware of the normal values for each of the vital signs and be proficient in the assessment of the values. The vital signs are normally taken as a series but will be discussed on an individual basis.

Blood Pressure

Blood pressure readings are created by the arterial pressure against the vessel wall. This is equivalent to the amount of pressure to push mercury in a sphygmomanometer on millimeter. This force is a result of the contractive phase of the left ventricle pushing blood into the aorta. At peak compression, the heart will have the maximum force. This is termed the systolic phase of the heart. During the process of ventricular relaxation, the pressure will drop to the minimal force; this phase is the diastolic phase. The blood pressure value is normally charted as systolic over diastolic values. The average blood pressure value is 120/80 mmHg. Hypertension occurs when a patient's systolic value is above 140, the diastolic value is above 90 mmHg, or both. Hypotension occurs when the systolic pressure is below 90 mmHg and only 60 mmHg in the diastolic phase.

Blood pressures are taken with the use of an aneroid or mercury manometer and a stethoscope. The aneroid manometer (blood pressure cuff) comes in a variety of sizes. The appropriate cuff should match the patient and body part. The technologist should always wash his or her hands before taking the patient's blood pressure. The patient should be positioned with the arm extended. Normally, blood pressure is taken with the cuff wrapped around the patient's arm, approximately 1 in. superior to the antecubital space. This places the cuff over the area of the brachial artery. The cuff should be wrapped snugly around the patient's arm, with the air valve open and the cuff deflated. The air valve should now be closed and the cuff inflated. As the cuff is inflated, the technologist should be able to palpate the brachial or radial artery. Inflation of the cuff should continue until the meter reads 30 mmHg above the point where the pulse disappears. The cuff should be deflated slowly by releasing the air valve. The technologist should note the point where the pulse becomes apparent. Continue to deflate the cuff and wait approximately 30 s to allow venous flow to prevent a false reading. The process is repeated with the diaphragm of the stethoscope placed over the brachial artery. Close the air valve, and reinflate the cuff to the level when 30 mmHg is above the systolic point. Slowly release the valve, allowing the mercury to fall at a rate of 2 to 3 mmHg/s. The systolic level is the point where the first clear pulsation sound appears. Continue releasing the cuff at the same rate until the pulsation sound disappears; this point is the diastolic level. Upon completion of the blood pressure readings, completely deflate and remove the cuff. Record the readings in the proper place on the chart and compare and evaluate the readings with previous levels and department standards.

Pulse

A pulse is present every time the left ventricle is contracted and forces blood into the arterial system. We can feel the presence of the pulse when we compress an artery against underlying muscle or bone structures. Pulse is frequently monitored on the medial side of the wrist in the area of the radial artery. When the body experiences a life-threatening situation, the body senses the need for the blood flow to the brain. This event may make the location of the pulse in the radial artery difficult. Other locations to monitor the pulse are the areas of the brachial, axilla, and carotid arteries. The peripheral blood circulation will usually decrease with an increase in life-threatening situations.

The technologist should wash his or her hands before taking the pulse of a patient. At the radial artery location, the technologist should place his or her thumb on the posterior side of the patient's wrist area. This method allows the technologist to place his or her fingers on the anterior side of the wrist over the radial artery. Lightly put pressure on the radial artery until the pulse is felt. Count the pulses for 15 s and then multiply the number of pulses by 4. This product will be the rate of pulse occurring in 1 min. The pulse rate should be charted and compared with the patient's normal rate or department standards. In addition, the pulse rate should be reported as normal, slow, rapid, weak, or irregular.

Respiration

Respiration is the normal exchange process occurring between the alveoli and red blood cells within the lungs. A visible full respiration cycle is from the point the patient has one complete inspiration and one complete expiration. When assessing the respiration of a patient, the technologist is assessing the breathing rate, depth, and rhythm. The process is charted as the number of cycles occurring in 1 min, whether the process involved shallow or normal breaths that were consistent or variable, and whether the respiration process was labored or not. Under normal conditions, it takes little conscious effort on the patient's part to complete the respiration process. When the patient has a noticeable effort in breathing, the technologist can visibly observe a pronounced movement of the neck, shoulders, and chest muscles. Checking respiration rate is normally a visual test, whereby the technologist inconspicuously observes the person breathing. This monitoring continues for 15 s, and the number of cycles is then multiplied by 4 to attain the number of cycles per minute. Checking respiration can be completed when checking the patient's pulse rate. The technologist should always be alert when there is a sudden change in a patient's respiration. Respiratory distress my occur when a patient has a sudden change in respiration rate, depth, or rhythm. In this event, the technologist should notify the physician.

Temperature

The normal temperature of the human body is 37°C (98.6°F). Exercise, disease, infection, or exposure to extreme warm or cold conditions can make temperatures occur above or below the normal value. Temperatures of patients in the diagnostic imaging department are normally checked orally. If the patient is at risk or unable to place a thermometer in the mouth, the option of an axillary measurement or tympanic-membrane measurement is possible. Current electronic thermometers are convenient and safe for oral and axillary monitoring of temperature. The technologist should be aware of the proper use of all thermometers kept in the facility.

CHAPTER 26

Quality Assurance Procedures

SIGNAL TO NOISE RATIO

Mandatory minimum required is 3.

Common Indications

- Quality assurance test to ensure the strongest possible signal within the capabilities of MR system.

Imaging Considerations

The signal is the usable voltage that has been induced in the receiver coil of the MRI unit. Background noise is within the signal and is contributed by the patient when placed within the bore of the magnet and also from inherent electrical noise of the MR unit itself. Noise is present at all frequencies and can be random. Signal to noise ratio (SNR) refers to the relationship of the amplitude of the received signal to the average amplitude of the noise. The signal is dependent on numerous factors, some of which can be altered. Common factors that can be adjusted to increase or decrease signal are proton density of the area of concern, flip angle, slice thickness, the number of times the information is sampled (NEX), the receive bandwidth, and type of receiver coil used. When considering methods of increasing SNR, there is usually a balance between image quality and scan time.

As part of the quality assurance procedure, the technologist should use the standard MR phantom to reference image quality. Phantoms are used to identify and evaluate artifacts within the MR image. The quality measurement should be taken each morning before the normal day of imaging. The results of this test should be compared throughout the month to monitor any change in the signal to noise ratio. Subtle changes can occur through items such as electrical interferences to the system.

CENTER FREQUENCY

Mandatory minimum required is 3.

Common Indications

- A method of calibration, which should be completed before acquisition
- Location of the central frequency of the transmitted RF pulse
- Determination of the effective RF amplitude to transmit

Imaging Considerations

For optimal image quality, the MR unit performs a precalibration test that ensures the MR unit will generate the ideal RF pulse, as well as the central frequency of the transmit bandwidth of the RF pulse. The precalibration process will also determine the magnitude of the transmitted RF pulse. The magnitude of the transmitted RF pulse should be sufficient to flip the hydrogen nuclei making up the net magnetic vector into the transverse plane. Distortion to images will occur if the magnitude of the RF pulse is too large. If the magnitude is too small, the signal to noise ratio is affected by the smaller generated signal. If the precalibration test fails, the technologist should inspect the coil and the connection between the coil ends. The precalibration test may also fail if the patient is too large or too small. In addition, precalibration may not function if the distribution of fat or water in the area to be saturated is uneven.

IMAGE PROCESSOR SENSITOMETRY

Mandatory minimum required is 3.

Common Indications

- To ensure the processor is functioning within the specified limits
- To ensure the processor is consistent and reproducible in image quality

Imaging Considerations

Sensitometry is a process using simulated light to expose film to a controlled set of light exposures, resulting in a step-wedge appearance with numerous shades of gray. Sensitometry is a quality assurance test used to evaluate a film's response to the exposure. Image processor sensitometry is a method to ensure that the processor will produce high-quality results consistently. Image processor sensitometry is one method of testing that assures the technologist that what we see on the monitor, as far as a quality diagnostic image, will appear similar on the film after processing has taken place. In the diagnostic imaging department, image processor sensitometry is commonly referred to as "running the strip."

Processor quality control is a daily exercise for MRI facilities, which uses dry processing or wet processing techniques for the developing film. For quality assurance of wet processors, it is likely your facility will have a "quality management" (QM) person within the department. Normally, this person is responsible for maintaining the tests concerning the quality assurance of the film processor. The QM person will have and maintain the acceptable quality standards associated with the specific processor. Processor quality control should be completed at minimum, before the day commences. To complete the image processor sensitometry for wet processors, the technologist will need a sensitometer, densitometer, and use of the same box of film set aside for quality assessment of the processor. The sensitometer exposes a radiographic film with an artificial light source. The resulting exposure from the sensitometer applies a gray scale image to the film. The film is processed, and the different shades of gray can be assessed with the use of a densitometer. The readings from the specified areas of the film are plotted and must fall in the category specified by the facility and manufacture. Differences in densities represent changes in contrast and speed. Depending on the department standards, the information from the sensitometry strips will be monitored and kept for the specified time. It is recommended the technologist contact the quality manager within the department to understand department standards in the area of image processor sensitometry.

Many MRI facilities use a method of laser printing and dry processing. This type of processor is linked to receive the image information from the MR host computer. Each time the dry processor is switched on, it will complete a systems check that is based on image quality. Depending on the model, this can occur after a time delay, when the processor has been left idle or when a new package of film has been loaded into the processor. The calibration test is to ensure that previous standards will be similar to those on the new sheet of film. The information received from the sensitometer will be stored within the processor's memory or printed out to meet the needs of the technologist or facility. The technologist must be confident the processor will produce consistent high-quality diagnostic images. If levels of acceptance are outside the standards set by the manufacturer and facility, either recalibration or service to the processor is needed.

EQUIPMENT INSPECTION
(e.g., COILS, CABLES, DOOR SEALS)

Mandatory minimum required is 3.

Common Indications

- Inspection of the coil to ensure a quality image and safety to the patient and technologist
- Inspection of the coil to ensure safety to the patient and technologist
- Inspection of the door and seal to ensure a quality image and safety to the patient and technologist

Imaging Considerations

Quality assurance involving coils, cables, and door seals means the technologist should inspect all three items throughout the course of the day. When imaging, coils should be inspected to be sure they are plugged in properly and the correct connector is used. The insulation around each cable should be inspected for signs of wear or fraying. Any coil displaying signs of wear should not be used. When imaging, the correct side of the coil should face the patient, with the coil placed close to the area of interest, without directly touching the skin. The coil may warm during the examination and result in patient concern or discomfort. To avoid this, placement of a positioning sponge or tissue between the coil and the patient's skin will insulate the contact area. Upon completion of the examination, the coil should be inspected before storage. Coils should be unplugged and removed from the bore of the magnet when not in use. The unplugged coil left within the bore of the magnet may absorb the energy simultaneously as the coil is being used. This can result in damaged coils and, more importantly, burns to the patient.

There are cables connected to coils and other components such as gating, triggering, and monitoring equipment. These electrical components associated with the use of MRI have been grounded and Faraday shielded to reduce the likelihood of RF energy affecting the cable. This is why only MR compatible components should be allowed within the imaging suite. When imaging, the cables should lay in a straight line manner to avoid looping. Loops of wire will conduct heat and result in patient discomfort or damage to the cable. All cables should be allowed to lay free of loops and, if possible, with something between the patient and cable such as a blanket or sheet.

The entrance to the MR suite should be established with only one possible entrance. The entrance door of the MR suite should display a warning sign regarding hazards of the magnetic field. Some imaging centers have a keyless security lock to prevent unauthorized personnel from entering the MR unit. The door entering the imaging room contains a locking mechanism that seals the door from unauthorized personnel and unauthorized RF influences. The door should remain closed during examination and when the MR unit is left unattended.

Bibliography

Agur, A.M. (1991) *Grant's Atlas of Anatomy*, 9th ed. Baltimore, MD: Williams & Wilkins.

Berquist, T.H. (1995) *Pocket Atlas of MRI Body Anatomy*, 2nd ed. Philadelphia, PA: Lippincott-Raven.

Bontrager, K.L. (1997) *Textbook of Radiographic Positioning and Related Anatomy*, 4th ed, (pp. 614–618). St. Louis, MO: Mosby.

Bushong, S.C. (1996) *Magnetic Resonance Imaging: Physical and Biological Principles*, 2nd ed, (pp. 329–428). St. Louis, MO: Mosby.

Computed Tomography Clinical Experience Requirements by the ARRT: Available at: http://www.arrt.org/ctsurvey.htm

Fishman, E.K. and Jeffrey, R.B. Jr. (eds) (1995) *Spiral CT Principles, Techniques, and Clinical Applications*. New York: Raven Press.

General Electric Company (1996) *Signa Horizon LX 1.5T Protocol Guide*. Milwaukee, WI: General Electric Co.

Haughton, V.M. and Daniels, D.L. (1986) *Pocket Atlas of Cranial Magnetic Resonance Imaging*. Philadelphia, PA: Lippincott-Raven.

Haus, A.G. and Jaskulski, S. M. (1997) *The Basics of Film Processing in Medical Imaging*. Madison, WI: Medical Physics Publishing.

Hendee, W.R. (1983) *The Physical Principles of Computed Tomography*. Boston, MA: Little, Brown and Company.

Kowalczyk, N. and Donnett, K. (1996) *Integrated Patient Care for the Imaging Professional* (pp. 111–262). St. Louis, MO: Mosby.

Lufkin, R.B. (1998) *The MRI Manual*, 2nd ed, (pp. 35–40). St. Louis, MO: Mosby.

Moss, A.A. (1992) *Interventional Computed Tomography*. In Moss, A.A. (ed), Gamsu, G., and Genant, H.K. *Computed Tomography of the Body with Magnetic Resonance Imaging* (Vol. 3, 2nd ed) Abdomen (pp.1297–1337). Philadelphia, PA: W.B. Saunders Company.

Newman, J. (1997) *Pharmacology for the Radiologic Technologist Parts 1,2,3*.

Pansky, B. (1984) *Review of Gross Anatomy*, 5th ed. New York: Macmillan.

Robb, R.A. (1996) Virtual computed endoscopy: Paper presented at the Visible human project conference, Oct. 7–8 1996, National Library of Medicine, National Institutes of Health, Bethesda, MD. Mayo Foundation/Clinic, Rochester, MN.

Silverman, P.M. (ed) (1998) *Helical (Spiral) Computed Tomography: A Practical Approach to Clinical Protocols*. Philadelphia, PA: Lippincott-Raven.

Thomas, C. L. (1993) *Taber's Cyclopedic Medical Dictionary*. Philadelphia, PA: F.A. Davis Company.

Torres, L.S. (1997) *Basic Medical Techniques and Patient Care for Radiologic Technologists*, 5th ed, (pp. 213–220). Philadelphia, PA: Lippincott-Raven.

Tortorici, M. (1992) *Concepts in Medical Radiographic Imaging, Circuitry, Exposure and Quality Control* (pp. 235–244). Philadelphia, PA: W.B. Saunders.

Vieco, R.T. (1995) *Helical/Spiral CT: A Practical Approach*. New York, NY: McGraw-Hill.

Vining, D.J., Liu, K., Choplin, R.H., Haponik, E.F. (1996) Virtual bronchoscopy: Relationships of virtual reality endobronchial simulations to actual bronchoscopic findings. *Chest* 109(5): 549.

Westbrook, C. (1994) *Handbook of MRI Technique*, Cambridge, MA: Blackwell Science, Inc.

Zeman, R.K., Brink, J.A., Costello, P., Davros, et al. (1995) *Helical/Spiral CT: A Practical Approach*. New York, NY: McGraw-Hill.

Suggestions from the Author:

It is suggested that the documentation of verifying officials include the name and address of the official. Comments should be clearly stated when necessary. It is important that simulated or elective examinations be noted. Any questions about competency verification should be directed to the body administering advanced certification.

Head
Routine Brain

Date completed	Facility name	Patient identification	Verifying official

*Ten competencies are required and *cannot* be simulated.

Head
Temporal Bone

Date completed	Facility name	Patient identification	Verifying official

*Five competencies are required.

Head
Orbit

Date completed	Facility name	Patient identification	Verifying official

*Five competencies are required.

Head
Sinuses

Date completed	Facility name	Patient identification	Verifying official

*Five competencies are required.

Head
Maxillofacial

Date completed	Facility name	Patient identification	Verifying official

*Five competencies are required.

Head
Pituitary

Date completed	Facility name	Patient identification	Verifying official

*Three competencies are *elective*.

Head
Temporomandibular Joint

Date completed	Facility name	Patient identification	Verifying official

*Three competencies are *elective*.

Head
Cerebral Angiography

Date completed	Facility name	Patient identification	Verifying official

*Three competencies are *elective*.

Neck
Soft Tissue

Date completed	Facility name	Patient identification	Verifying official

*Five competencies are mandatory.

Neck
Larynx

Date completed	Facility name	Patient identification	Verifying official

*Three competencies are *elective*.

Neck
Carotid Angiography

Date completed	Facility name	Patient identification	Verifying official

*Three competencies are *elective*.

Spine
Cervical

Date completed	Facility name	Patient identification	Verifying official

*Five competencies are mandatory.

Spine
Lumbosacral

Date completed	Facility name	Patient identification	Verifying official

*Five competencies are mandatory.

Spine
Post Myelography

Date completed	Facility name	Patient identification	Verifying official

*Three competencies are *elective*.

Spine
Thorasic

Date completed	Facility name	Patient identification	Verifying official

*Three competencies are *elective*.

Chest
Mediastinum

Date completed	Facility name	Patient identification	Verifying official

*Ten competencies are required and *cannot* be simulated.

Chest
Vascular (Heart and Great Vessels)

Date completed	Facility name	Patient identification	Verifying official

*Five competencies are required.

Chest
Lung

Date completed	Facility name	Patient identification	Verifying official

*Five competencies are required.

Chest
High-Resolution CT

Date completed	Facility name	Patient identification	Verifying official

*Five competencies are required.

Abdomen and Pelvis

Date completed	Facility name	Patient identification	Verifying official

*Ten competencies are required and *cannot* be simulated.

Abdomen and Pelvis
Liver

Date completed	Facility name	Patient identification	Verifying official

*Five competencies are required.

Abdomen and Pelvis
Pancreas

Date completed	Facility name	Patient identification	Verifying official

*Five competencies are required.

Abdomen and Pelvis
Kidneys

Date completed	Facility name	Patient identification	Verifying official

*Five competencies are required.

Abdomen and Pelvis
Vascular

Date completed	Facility name	Patient identification	Verifying official

*Five competencies are required.

Abdomen and Pelvis
Routine Pelvis

Date completed	Facility name	Patient identification	Verifying official

*Five competencies are required.

Abdomen and Pelvis
Adrenals

Date completed	Facility name	Patient identification	Verifying official

*Three competencies are *elective*.

Abdomen and Pelvis
GI Tract

Date completed	Facility name	Patient identification	Verifying official

*Three competencies are *elective*.

Musculoskeletal
Upper Extremity

Date completed	Facility name	Patient identification	Verifying official

*Five competencies are required.

Musculoskeletal
Lower Extremity

Date completed	Facility name	Patient identification	Verifying official

*Five competencies are required.

Musculoskeletal
Pelvic Girdle (Hips)

Date completed	Facility name	Patient identification	Verifying official

*Five competencies are required and *cannot* be simulated.

Musculoskeletal
Post-Arthrography

Date completed	Facility name	Patient identification	Verifying official

*Three competencies are elective.

Interventional Procedures (Includes Evaluation of any Lab Values)
Biopsy

Date completed	Facility name	Patient identification	Verifying official

*Three competencies are required and *cannot* be simulated.

Interventional Procedures (Includes Evaluation of Lab Values)
Drainage

Date completed	Facility name	Patient identification	Verifying official

*Three competencies are *elective* but *cannot* be simulated.

Interventional Procedures (Includes Evaluation of Lab Values)
Aspiration

Date completed	Facility name	Patient identification	Verifying official

*Three competencies are *elective* but *cannot* be simulated.

Interventional Procedures
Portography

Date completed	Facility name	Patient identification	Verifying official

*Three competencies are *elective* but *cannot* be simulated.

Special Procedures
Leg Length

Date completed	Facility name	Patient identification	Verifying official

*Three competencies are *elective* and *cannot* be simulated.

Special Procedures
Pelvimetry

Date completed	Facility name	Patient identification	Verifying official

*Three competencies are *elective* and *cannot* be simulated.

Special Procedures
Radiation Therapy Planning

Date completed	Facility name	Patient identification	Verifying official

*Three competencies are *elective* and *cannot* be simulated.

Special Procedures
Spiral

Date completed	Facility name	Patient identification	Verifying official

*Five competencies are *elective* and *cannot* be simulated.

Special Procedures
Stereotaxis

Date completed	Facility name	Patient identification	Verifying official

*Three competencies are *elective* and *cannot* be simulated.

Special Procedures
Pediatric Imaging (6 Years or Younger)

Date completed	Facility name	Patient identification	Verifying official

*Five competencies are *elective* and *cannot* be simulated.

Special Procedures
Nonincremental Dynamic Scanning

Date completed	Facility name	Patient identification	Verifying official

*Three procedures are *elective*.

Special Procedures
Post-Processing Multiplanar Reconstruction

Date completed	Facility name	Patient identification	Verifying official

*Five competencies are required.

Special Procedures
Post-Processing 3-D Vascular Reconstruction

Date completed	Facility name	Patient identification	Verifying official

*Five competencies are *elective*.

Special Procedures
Post-Processing 3-D Bone Reconstruction

Date completed	Facility name	Patient identification	Verifying official

*Five competencies are *elective*.

Special Procedures
Fly Through Navigator Post-Processing

Date completed	Facility name	Patient identification	Verifying official

*Three competencies are *elective* but *cannot* be simulated.

Patient Care
Vital Signs (Hemodynamic Monitoring, Respiration, Pulse Oximetry, and Temperature)

Date completed	Facility name	Patient identification	Verifying official

*Five competencies are required.

Patient Care
Universal Precautions

Date completed	Facility name	Patient identification	Verifying official

*Five competencies are required.

Patient Care
Oxygen Administration

Date completed	Facility name	Patient identification	Verifying official

*Three competencies are required.

Patient Care
Assessment and Monitoring of Consciousness and Respiration**

Date completed	Facility name	Patient identification	Verifying official

*Five competencies are required.
**See Glasgow Coma Scale.

Patient Care
Assessment and Contraindications for Procedure

Date completed	Facility name	Patient identification	Verifying official

*Five competencies are required.

Patient Care
Sterile Technique

Date completed	Facility name	Patient identification	Verifying official

*Three competencies are required.

Patient Care
Verification of Informed Consent (When Necessary)

Date completed	Facility name	Patient identification	Verifying official

*Three competencies are required.

Patient Care
CPR Certification

Date completed	Facility name	Verifying official

Contrast Administration (IV, Oral, Rectal, or Catheter)
Evaluation of Lab Values Prior to Procedure

Date completed	Facility name	Patient identification	Verifying official

*Five competencies are required.

Contrast Administration (IV, Oral, Rectal, or Catheter)
Contrast Agent Selection

Date completed	Facility name	Patient identification	Verifying official

*Five competencies are required.

Contrast Administration
Contrast Agent Preparation

Date completed	Facility name	Patient identification	Verifying official

*Five competencies are required.

Contrast Administration
Site Selection

Date completed	Facility name	Patient identification	Verifying official

*Five competencies are required.

Contrast Administration
Venipuncture

Date completed	Facility name	Patient identification	Verifying official

*Five competencies are required and *can* be *simulated* in states or institutions.
  Prohibit venipuncture by a registered technologist.

Contrast Administration
Power Injection (Loading, Selecting Rate, and Emergency Stop)

Date completed	Facility name	Patient identification	Verifying official

*Five competencies are required.

Contrast Administration
Monitoring Patients for Adverse Reactions

Date completed	Facility name	Patient identification	Verifying official

*Five competencies are required.

Functions for Image Display
Geometric Measurement

Date completed	Facility name	Patient identification	Verifying official

*Five competencies are required.

Functions for Image Display
ROI

Date completed	Facility name	Patient identification	Verifying official

*Five competencies are required.

Functions for Image Display
Target/Zoom

Date completed	Facility name	Patient identification	Verifying official

*Five competencies are mandatory.

369

Functions for Image Display
Histograms

Date completed	Facility name	Patient identification	Verifying official

*Three competencies are *elective*.

Functions for Image Display
Highlighting

Date completed	Facility name	Patient identification	Verifying official

*Three competencies are *elective*.

Quality Assurance Procedures
Calibration (Using Appropriate Phantom)

Date completed	Facility name	Patient identification	Verifying official

*Five competencies are required.

Quality Assurance Procedures
CT Number

Date completed	Facility name	Patient identification	Verifying official

*Five competencies are required.

Quality Assurance Procedures
Noise

Date completed	Facility name	Patient identification	Verifying official

*Five competencies are required.

Quality Assurance Procedures
Linearity

Date completed	Facility name	Patient identification	Verifying official

*Three procedures are *elective*.

Quality Assurance Procedures
Spatial Resolution

Date completed	Facility name	Patient identification	Verifying official

*Three competencies are *elective*.

Quality Assurance
Contrast Resolution

Date completed	Facility name	Patient identification	Verifying official

*Three competencies are *elective*.

Head and Neck
Brain

Date completed	Facility name	Patient identification	Verifying official

*Ten competencies are required.

Head and Neck
Internal Auditory Canal

Date completed	Facility name	Patient identification	Verifying official

*Four competencies are required.

Head and Neck
Pituitary

Date completed	Facility name	Patient identification	Verifying official

*Four competencies are required.

Head and Neck
Orbit

Date completed	Facility name	Patient identification	Verifying official

*Four competencies are required.

Head and Neck
Vascular Imaging

Date completed	Facility name	Patient identification	Verifying official

*Four competencies are required.

Head and Neck
Cranial Nerves

Date completed	Facility name	Patient identification	Verifying official

*Three competencies are *elective*.

Head and Neck
Soft Tissue Neck

Date completed	Facility name	Patient identification	Verifying official

*Three competencies are *elective*.

Spine
Cervical

Date completed	Facility name	Patient identification	Verifying official

*Ten competencies are required.

Spine
Thoracic

Date completed	Facility name	Patient identification	Verifying official

*Six competencies are required.

Spine
Lumbosacral

Date completed	Facility name	Patient identification	Verifying official

*Ten competencies are required.

Thorax
Brachial Plexus

Date completed	Facility name	Patient identification	Verifying official

*Three competencies are *elective*.

Thorax
Mediastinum

Date completed	Facility name	Patient identification	Verifying official

*Three competencies are *elective*.

Thorax
Vascular Imaging/Great Vessels

Date completed	Facility name	Patient identification	Verifying official

*Three competencies are *elective*.

Thorax
Heart

Date completed	Facility name	Patient identification	Verifying official

*Three competencies are *elective*.

Thorax
Breast

Date completed	Facility name	Patient identification	Verifying official

*Three competencies are *elective*.

Abdomen and Pelvis
Liver, Pancreas, or Spleen

Date completed	Facility name	Patient identification	Verifying official

*Four competencies are required and one of each must be done.

Abdomen and Pelvis
Pelvis

Date completed	Facility name	Patient identification	Verifying official

*Four competencies are required.

Abdomen and Pelvis
Kidneys

Date completed	Facility name	Patient identification	Verifying official

*Three competencies are *elective*.

Abdomen and Pelvis
Adrenals

Date completed	Facility name	Patient identification	Verifying official

*Three competencies are *elective*.

Abdomen and Pelvis
Vascular Imaging

Date completed	Facility name	Patient identification	Verifying official

*Three competencies are *elective*.

Abdomen and Pelvis
Prostate

Date completed	Facility name	Patient identification	Verifying official

*Three competencies are *elective*.

Musculoskeletal
Shoulder

Date completed	Facility name	Patient identification	Verifying official

*Six competencies are required.

Musculoskeletal
Elbow, Wrist, or Hand

Date completed	Facility name	Patient identification	Verifying official

*Four competencies, in any combination, are required.

Musculoskeletal
Hip

Date completed	Facility name	Patient identification	Verifying official

*Four competencies are required.

Musculoskeletal
Knee

Date completed	Facility name	Patient identification	Verifying official

*Six competencies are required.

Musculoskeletal
Ankle or Foot

Date completed	Facility name	Patient identification	Verifying official

*Four competencies are required.

Musculoskeletal
Temporomandibular Joint

Date completed	Facility name	Patient identification	Verifying official

*Three competencies are elective.

Musculoskeletal
Long Bone

Date completed	Facility name	Patient identification	Verifying official

*Three competencies are *elective*.

Musculoskeletal
Pelvic Girdle

Date completed	Facility name	Patient identification	Verifying official

*Three competencies are *elective*.

Musculoskeletal
Vascular Imaging

Date completed	Facility name	Patient identification	Verifying official

*Three competencies are *elective*.

Musculoskeletal
Kinematic Studies

Date completed	Facility name	Patient identification	Verifying official

*Three competencies are *elective*.

Advanced Imaging Procedures
Perfusion/Diffusion Imaging

Date completed	Facility name	Patient identification	Verifying official

*Three competencies are *elective*.

Advanced Imaging Procedures
Functional MRI (fMRI)

Date completed	Facility name	Patient identification	Verifying official

*Three competencies are *elective*.

Advanced Imaging Procedures
Echo Planar Imaging (EPI)

Date completed	Facility name	Patient identification	Verifying official

*Three competencies are *elective*.

Advanced Imaging Procedures
3-D Volume Reformation

Date completed	Facility name	Patient identification	Verifying official

*Three competencies are *elective*.

Advanced Imaging Procedures
Multiplanar Reformation

Date completed	Facility name	Patient identification	Verifying official

*Three competencies are *elective*.

Advanced Imaging Procedures
Spectroscopy

Date completed	Facility name	Patient identification	Verifying official

*Three competencies are *elective*.

Patient Care Procedures
Contrast Media Preparation

Date completed	Facility name	Patient identification	Verifying official

*Four competencies are required.

Patient Care Procedures
Venipuncture

Date completed	Facility name	Patient identification	Verifying official

*Four competencies are required but may be simulated in states or institutions, which
  prohibit registered technologists from performing venipucture.

Patient Care Procedures
Vital Signs (Pulse, Respiration, Temperature, Blood Pressure)

Date completed	Facility name	Patient identification	Verifying official

*Four competencies are required.

Patient Care Procedures
CPR Certification

Date completed	Facility name	Verifying official

*Must be within 24 months preceding application for advanced examination.

Quality Assurance
Signal to Noise

Date completed	Facility name	Patient identification	Verifying official

*Three competencies are required.

Quality Assurance
Center Frequency

Date completed	Facility name	Patient identification	Verifying official

*Three competencies are required.

Quality Assurance
Image Processor Sensitometry

Date completed	Facility name	Patient identification	Verifying official

*Three competencies are required.

Quality Assurance
Equipment Inspection (Coils, Cables, Door Seals, Etc.)

Date completed	Facility name	Patient identification	Verifying official

*Three competencies are required.